GET TO KNOW YOUR TEENAGER
UNDERSTANDING HOW THEY TALK

Written by:

A teacher and a psychologist
N. De la Puerta and Borja Núñez
Teens'Detectives

DOBLETINTA EDITORIAL

ISBN: 9798871043219

DOBLETINTA

DEDICATION

"To my parents and my children, my students and teachers, and to everyone who has taught me something in life. Thank you".

"To Sonia. To Thaly. To Greece".

CONTENT

"The limits of my language are the limits of my mind."
LUDWIG WITTGENSTEIN.

INTRODUCTION

"*Das lache,*" my eldest son, now a teenager, told me as he retired to his room so as not to have to watch the little victory dance I was dedicating to him. After several very painful defeats, in which one observes in bewilderment how the children begin to beat the father without the father feigning defeat for the children, he had finally managed to defeat him.eitherto FIFA.

I was so happy for the victory, so dedicated to my dance, that at that moment I did not notice that expression. But the next morning, before preparing to do some exercises to consolidate what we had seen about the French Revolution and the American War of Independence, it occurred to me to ask my students the question that I should have asked my son: "By the way, What does *dar lache* mean?" I asked without further ado. There was a brief, bewildered silence. "Why? In what context, teacher?" Ricardo dared to say. "My son told me yesterday that he gave lache," I responded. Again, there was silence, but this time much longer and more uncomfortable, a silence accompanied by telltale glances that they gave each other, at me out of the corner of their eye.. Msome of them jokey, others full of pitiful empathy for my situation.

"*Dar lache* is the same as giving cringe." Finally, Carmen took pity on me enough to break the silence. Always Carmen, always above what others will say. It caught my attention that such a reserved girl was the one who always broke the ice, fearlessly exposing herself to her classmates while the others remained silent, protected in the crowd. Later I would understand this way of being, the reason for her reservations, but understand that I cannot share that story with you. That story is Carmen's story.

"And what is cringe? Forgive my ignorance, but I still don't understand," I apologized sincerely, overwhelmed by the surprised faces that filled the classroom. "Well, basically, you're a jerk, teacher," Manuel replied amused. "No, that's not it. Lache and cringearetheway of saying"Now what those of your age call other people's shame" Valeria defined with the usual neatness and lack of tact typical of her youth.

That finally resolved my doubt, but it raised many others in me: Was my son ashamed of me? How could I communicate with him as he grew older if I didn't understand him? How could he maintain the respect of my students if he showed such ignorance of their slang? PerhapstheWhat did I think highly of when they showed they didn't know everything I had explained to them for months or when they did so by bathing the scant data in a sea of spelling mistakes and grammatical errors? How could I help youeitheryesto growif it was so difficult for me to get to know himeitheryes? And the question that struck me the most at that moment: Had Manuel wanted to make me understand what my son felt by telling me that he was upset, or on the contrary had he taken advantage of my confusion to sneak in a veiled insult? How many times does the lack of definition, ambiguity or radical changes of adolescents leave us with this type of doubt, in which we do not know whether to act with severity, exercising our role as educators, mothers or fathers, or let it run and look for on the other hand due to the possibility of misinterpretation. In this case, I don't know if I was right or not, Manuel escapedof reprimand.

I posed these same questions (except for Manuel's, which I reserved until telling you now) to Borja Núñez, an experienced psychologist who was also bitten by the bug to practically corroborate what he knew in theory about adolescent slang. And these and many other questions that arose and that inspired us to investigate like detectives and write this book with the answers to what we have discovered, which we hope can be useful to you. In our case, that's how it was. Although I cannot tell you Carmen's story, I must tell you that I was able to get to know her much better and we were able to work on her problems, a complicated situation that was very difficult for her to verbalize to anyone, as it generated a natural distrust of everyone. By understanding her language and figuring out how to use it, we got her to open up. And this is something very complex, since it is not about knowing and using their slang, but about knowing how to use it in times and ways that allow us to get close enough to know them, knowing how to interpret in advance the different semantic fields in which they are pronounced, that vary depending on context. Knowing them, in short, either because they speak to us directly (rarely, since they don't even know each other enough to express it yet), or because we can stay close to them long enough to study and understand what they do and, above all, what they do. what do they say. A complex investigation, which personally is being very useful to me in my relationship with my children and inheI work with my students and now we want to share with you to help youeitherHe knows how to deepen the bond with his daughters and sons, help himeitherknows how to know them better and therefore, to guide them better, and to be able to anticipate possible risks in their environment before they experience them. In short, a guide that helps you enjoy them much more in a stage in which each new thing seems to surpass us at times. That is the objective of Teens' Detectives: discreet and in-depth investigation at the service of mothers and fathers of teenagers. We hope that this book and the upcoming research we publish will be useful to you.

1. TEENAGE SLANG

Until that moment, I did not remember a greater joy than the one I felt when Sonia, my wife, gave me the long-awaited news: We were going to be parents! As a responsible and cultured person that I consider myself to be, I dedicated the months of pregnancy to reading everything that fell into my power about the moment of childbirth, the puerperium and the upbringing of the child (a boy, they confirmed to us) who was about to appear in our lives.

In those first years, with each crisis that arose, whether the baby's own or our existential ones, there was always a text with the keys to solving them: breastfeeding crisis, the first teeth, the first tantrums, the fears... It seemed that we were capable to control the situation, so, in a display of bravery, we set out to look for a second child, who soon arrived. And even in a display of unconsciousness, a third arrived. Everything has been going more or less well for us until recently. Aside from the difficulties that come with going through life with a large family, things continued their course, the course set out in the parenting guides. Until one day...

Nobody warned us. We didn't see it written in any guide. One night you put a sweet, adorable child to bed and the next morning you wake up a hairy, grumpy teenager, who greets you with a couple of shouts for waking him up so early. Adolescence does not follow "the written course." He appears overnight, without the progressive evolution of him and without you even having time to drink coffee to assimilate it.

Today, both Sonia and I, the situation seems more controlled. Don't worry, we haven't gone for the room. With three children we feel that our happiness is overflowing... and our patience, and our energies, and... And how have we managed to feel more confident? We have simply recycled the obsolete guides for parents, we have tried to convey all the love we feel and we have taken the edge off of adolescent crises, because for them everything is transcendent and at the same time, everything changes abruptly. There is no healthy mind that can withstand that intensity and those ups and downs if it is not taking them less seriously and with more humor.

It is fun to see how the physical changes they experience are accompanied by aesthetic changes, in an attempt to recognize themselves, to find their identity in that sea of transformations in which they often drown if they do not have someone nearby who loves them and who I threw them a lifeline. When you become obsessed with one of those aesthetic changes that we find difficult to accept, but that we end up accepting, I recommend taking as many photos as you can of the moment. Their outbursts are much better tolerated when we understand the difficulty of the process they go through and when we have ammunition for our little personal revenge, to use once they pass that stage and threaten the next one.

Among the many changes they incorporate into their lives, using a coded language that allows them to communicate with their peers without being detected by their elders is one of the most significant. Regardless of where in the world they live, the historical moment in which they find themselves, Adolescents develop their own language. Your Slang.

Teen slang is a form of communication that goes beyond common words and phrases. It shows that process of constructing your identity that we mentioned before, and that we would like to help you with.eitherYou can decipher it with this book. A slow process, which builds little by little, as their slang provides them with what they need. But,what do they need?

First, creating unique slang allows them to feel part of a group. By using it, adolescents seek to establish necessary meaningful connections with their peers. It allows them, therefore, to begin to define themselves.

Furthermore, the adoption of slang is also a form of subtle rebellion. Adolescents seek to separate themselves from adult authority to establish their own identity. Using Slang that adults do not understand is a way to establish a communication barrier and assert your independence. It allows them, therefore, to create the necessary space in which they can continue to define themselves.

Finally, slang can allow teens to talk about sensitive or uncomfortable topics covertly. This gives them a space to discuss personal or controversial topics without feeling judged. That is, it gives them the necessary freedom to make the decisions that will end up defining them.

This is a natural, necessary process that is repeated regardless of the historical stage in which we find ourselves. We live it too. But what is a natural and healthy process can turn into a nightmare when in that space of freedom that they have built, in which connections with their peers are so relevant, they lead them to make decisions that are harmful to them. Knowing their Slang, understanding what they say, can help us detect where the risks come from and allows us to address them preventively.

Do we mean by this that we should allow teenagers to speak their slang whenever they feel like it? No Please! Not at all.

"Teacher, you've taken me away here and I have the answer right," Diego told me when reviewing the exams. He had lowered him a few tenths on a question in which, in fact, he was not wrong in substance, although he was wrong in form. "Of course, Diego. You cannot write in an exam that the changes of the industrial revolution came to Spain with a lot of lag. There are contexts in which you cannot speak as you want, but as you must." "F," he responded in a brief statement, but one that suggested that he accepted the correction.

I understood those terms, since they are related to the world of computing and video games of which I have some notions. He knew that lag is a term that refers to the excessive delay that occurs between sending data and receiving it (in that sense, he nailed the statement about Spanish industrialization in the 19th century). He also knew the expression F, he had heard it from other kids before. It was originally born in the game Call of Duty and is used as support or empathy towards someone facing a difficult moment or, as in this case, to express sadness at the difficult moment itself.

In this case, the lesson that Diego had to learn was not about History. And I also learned a lot from this conversation. I got to know Diego better, an extraordinary boy, indeed very fond of computers and video games, but capable of balancing his passion with his responsibilities as a student and without neglecting his friendships, which makes him very loved. Of course, as in this case, sometimes he is somewhat impulsive. I am convinced that the nerves before the exam, together with the frequent use of these terms, which are part of their normal language (since there is no way for them to get used to checking their answers before handing in),atest), they played a trick on him. Although it is important to allow adolescents to express themselves in their own Slang for everything it gives them (and for everything it can give us to get to know our son or daughter who is defining themselves), it is equally important to correct them when the context or the situation are not appropriate. Teenagers must learn how to adapt their language to communicate effectively.

We usually teach this, but it is harder for us to learn. When we talk to them, we tend to demand communication on our terms, in our language, without showing respect for theirs. And this means that communication often breaks down. It is not about talking like teenagers at our age, we will go into more detail about it later. It's about showing interest in what matters to them. Be close, because when we speak closely, shouting is not necessary and communication becomes possible. With Diego himselfI hadmany other conversations, some very personal related to the sentimental situations that he was beginning to experience, in which he needed to use his usual expressions to be able to describe his emotions, and in which it was good for me to use some of them myself to show the necessary empathy. .

There are many terms that are part of adolescent slang. Terms also evolve, fall into disuse or are enriched with new meanings. It often includes concepts that are unique to a generation, based on cultural references, music, trends and technology of the moment. These terms can change quickly as new fads and trends emerge, keeping the slang fresh and relevant for today's teens. We must also not forget that since it is related to the context in which it is handled, it varies greatly from one place to another. The task of gathering all the terms spoken in the world and also keeping them updated seems simply unbearable to us. But in our research, we have specified well-differentiated semantic fields, which are shared by everyone, regardless of where they live, which we have called sources of linguistic influence. We have based ourselves on Spanish slang (the closest to us) and English-speaking slang (the most widespread) to exemplify them.

These sources of linguistic influence are the following:
- **Video game.**
- **Social networks.**
- **Visual elements.**
- **Popular music.**
- **Risk situations.**

If you like, in honor of Diego, we will start with the first one.

2. VIDEO GAME SLANG

When you have children, there are unique, very special moments in which we can almost see how they grow before our eyes: when they say their first word, when they take their first step, when they get their first tooth... or when they ask you for their first gaming headset. and a killing game. That was what our son Dani told us when we asked him what he would be excited for us to give him on one of his last birthdays. Well, he didn't say "killing game," he said Fornite, but to my wife and I it sounded like he had directly asked us for an assault rifle. Looking at it today, I think we exaggerated a little, but of course, we were used to him asking us for things about dinosaurs or Pokémon and the change came completely unexpectedly. That was one of those moments when we saw before our eyes how our son was growing up. A teenager had been born.

The time left until his birthday was very good for us to investigate a little about this new reality in which our son, for the first time, was ahead. It is a constant for parents of teenagers to have to make decisions about topics about which we only have a few notions, which also tend to be negative, since we have learned about them through channels that we do know, such as the press and radio programs or television, which tend to treat them with sensational overtones, or anecdotes told by other parents, whose interest iseitherIt lies in the fact that they are not going to end well. Nobody says "well, they gave Fortnite to my neighbor's son and now he gets very good grades and has many friends." If we change good for bad and many for few, it surely comes close to some of the conversations we have had so many times with other mothers and fathers.

With many more doubts than certainties, I could not avoid the temptation of consulting my particular committee of experts. It coincided in time with the agenda ofggeographyandeconomic, specifically the primary sector, which, honestly, is difficult to sharpen so that it is received with the enthusiasm that one always aspires to achieve. As expected,nor I was getting it, at least they didn't show the same enthusiasm that I did receive when I proposed this short break for the consultation. "Hey, teacher, you're a noob. You have no idea. But if Fornite isn't a shooter, younger kids can play perfectly," said Paula. "What happens is that he is a boomer, but at least he works with his children," said Sergio, who I hope does not end up being a lawyer with similar defenses. "In Fortnite you don't need to kill, just survive," Ricardo clarified to me. "Yes, but camping, and that""ugly" Mateo messed with me again. A great stir was generated, with multiple interventions in which those whose experience in video games was enormous (and did not understand my doubts) were mixed, and those who complained of having excessively restrictive parents, who did not let them play. as they would like (and they didn't understand my doubts either). The interventions of Paula and Sergio especially caught my attention, because of the vehemence with which they talked about video games and, above all, because they are both wonderful people, as students they have very different profiles. Let's say, without naming names, that one of them is not a model student. His grades could be improved and he is not known for his proactivity or waste of his efforts. Sergio, however, has excellent grades, and stands out for making an effort to learn and not beingeitherit in approving. This caught my attention a lot. He tended to prejudge the consumption of video games with poor performance in academic grades, but this was not the case for Sergio. Would he be an exception or was he wrong?

When I mentioned it to Borja, Sergio's profile did not surprise him at all. His training and experience as a psychologist made him have a much broader and clearer vision than I did, but my doubts seemed significant to him, because in his opinion, they were those that any mother or father could have. So finding answers to my questions was the starting point of our research, which we will begin to break down below.

Before trying to decipher the meaning of gamer Slang, it is important to know the different types of games that exist, since it will be very useful for us to know the tastes of our children to begin to discover them in this aspect of theirs. We have defined eleven basic types, each with a different play style, objectives, intensity level and lingo.

Third Person Shooter (TPS):
Shooting game in which the point of view is a camera behind the character you control.

First Person Shooter (FPS):
Shooting game that places you inside the character you control.

MMO:
A massively multiplayer game, where hundreds or thousands of players share the same world online.

RPG:
A single-player role-playing game, where you level up a character over time to take on more powerful enemies.

MMORPG:
A massively multiplayer online role-playing game.

MOBA:
Online Multiplayer Battlefield: A highly competitive game, in which you have to command a single protagonist who is part of an online team.

RTS:
Real time strategy games. They are tactical action with a fast pace.

SIM:
Simulation games of real experiences, such as racing or flying.

CCG:
Collectible card games. They are digital versions of classic card games.

4X:
In English, eXplore, eXpand, eXploit, eXterminate. They are strategy games where the objective is to conquer the world.

Sandbox:
Offline games, with an open world that you can explore freely.

To find out the Slang used in each one, the most fun thing was to go directly to the source: the gamers. We can find a multitude of videos starring teenagers (and not so teenagers), who comment while playing the game, speaking in an encrypted language. They are known as casters. When I watch any of his videos, the feeling is that of a traveler interacting with people from exotic and unknown worlds. Then the mirror makes it clear to me that I have only gotten older. Time Traveler, at least.

From the research that Borja and I have carried out, we have selected those terms that seem most relevant to us, either because they are frequently used, or because they are associated with video games that may make us more suspicious, such as those about killing (shooter) or that are played with other unknown online players (MMO). As in the rest of this guide, we are going to select the most used in Spanish and the most frequent in English, although in this case, many are shared, since in Spanish they tend to use terms derived from, if not the same as, English.

Most common terms of video game slang in Spanish:

1S1K:
Acronym for the English 1 Shot 1 Kill (one shot, one death). Kill an enemy with a single shot.
Ban:
From the English ban (forbid). Blocking access, generally to a service or an online game server. Having a ban or Being banned means having access to a service, server, forum, etc. blocked.
Buged:
Colloquial expression to indicate that a game or a part of it has bugs (errors) that prevent its correct functioning.
Camp:
Camping.
Camping:
From English, camping (camp). In multiplayer games, it is a tactic that consists of remaining motionless at a strategic point on the map that is difficult to access or has poor visibility, waiting for other players to appear in line of fire to shoot them. It is a very frowned upon strategy and is even penalized on

some servers.

Carry:

Derived from Carry. When a player "runs" it means that he has enough skill or power to make his team win on his own.

Cast:

1. From English cast (throw). Cast spells.

2. From English cast (to emit). Publish videos, live or recorded, of competitive video game games commenting on their development.

Caster:

1. From English caster (caster). Character or player who has the ability to use magic or ranged attack spells.

2. Person who "casts" (broadcasts) videos of competitive video games with comments.

Chetado:

1. Said of a player who is using cheats (tricks) to have an advantage in the game.

2. Said of a character, skill, object, weapon, etc. which is too powerful compared to the rest, poorly balanced. Synonym of broken.

Chinese Farmer:

Vulgar way of referring to people who dedicate themselves to playing many hours of online games in exchange for a salary, or other compensation such as accommodation and food, in order to raise characters to a certain level, generally to the maximum level, so that later These are sold to players who do not want to invest the time necessary to level up a character.

This practice emerged in China (hence the term), but it is common anywhere in the world to find people who use these types of practices to make money.

Counter peeking:

From English to peek (take a look) and counter (against). In first-person shooting games, the action of repeatedly peeking out (to seek vision of the rival at a crossfire angle) and returning to cover, taking advantage of this moment to return to shoot.

Craft:

From English craft (to elaborate). Make objects from existing ones or from basic elements collectible in a game. It is a very common skill in role-playing games.

Dupe:

From the English dupe (to deceive). Taking advantage of an error or glitch in the game to obtain successive duplicates or clones of an item, to use it indefinitely or to sell it.

Epicity:

It comes from epic, that is, great or out of the ordinary, in reference to a game, game, specific action, etc.

Gank:

Do ganking.

Ganking:

Acronym for Gang Killing.

In massively online games, a practice in which a group of players moves around the game world to eliminate other lone players, usually from other factions or guilds.

It can also refer to the same practice, but carried out by a single player on other players of a much lower level than his own.

Ghosting:

From English ghost (ghost). In online multiplayer games, watch the stream (broadcast of the game) of the opposing team at the same time as it is being played, which allows you to play with an advantage by knowing the opponent's actions.

Grind:

Spanishization of the English term grinding (to grind, to crush). Killing enemies repeatedly with the sole objective of accumulating some reward, such as experience to level up a character or some equipment or materials.

Hater:

Derived from the English to hate (hate) / hater (he who hates). Player who systematically despises, destructively criticizes or defames a game, genre, brand, platform, etc.

It differs from the troll in that it does not generally seek to attract attention.

Kappa:

Emoticon or meme used at the end of a sentence to indicate that it is ironic or sarcastic, commonly used on the streaming platform Twitch.

Kilombear:

In Argentina, synonymous with interrupting, spoiling, bothering, etc. in a game.

Laged:
Equivalent to "having lag", that is, having such a great delay in communication with the server and/or the rest of the players in a game that it becomes very difficult or directly impossible to play an online video game correctly.

Lick:
From English lamer (in computer slang, an ignorant person). Performing actions typical of a lick, that is, behaving stupidly, cheating or annoying others, and ultimately in a state of ignorance about the correct way to play.
In certain video games it can have a more specific meaning, but always in reference to stupid, cheating or annoying behavior for other players.

Literated:
From English lit (illuminated). Used mainly in shooting games, a teammate is called "liteado" to finish off an enemy who has been injured after a confrontation.

LOL:
1. Acronym for League of Legends, a MOBA-type online real-time strategy video game developed by Riot Games in 2009.
2. Acronym for the English expression Laughing out Loud, very commonly used on the Internet.

One-armed:
Extremely bad player, due to inexperience or lack of playing ability.

Rat Boy:
Young person, generally pre-adolescent, who tries to appear rude, despite his or her young age, through shouting, insults and generally hostile behavior, which is usually extremely noisy, exaggerated and tiring.
In the field of online video games, this is usually called all those kids who, due to their young age, have a very strident voice and who spend most of their time shouting into the microphone, often playing video games that are not appropriate for their age. .

Noob:
From English newbie (newbie). Derogatory way of referring to a rookie, generally for not respecting older players, or for not improving over time.

Chicken:

In shooting games or shooters, a player who dies too many times.

Ratear:

Similar to camping, being hidden or camouflaged, aiming at your rival from afar to try to kill him.

Rekt:

From the English rekt, vulgarism of wrecked (crushed, destroyed). Rekt or Get Rekt is a vulgar expression, common among young people and adolescents, to provoke the player or the opposing team, as a synonym for "We are going to crush/destroy you."

Roleplay:

Role (role, function). Play according to the rules and characteristics of a role-playing game or simply play a role-playing game.

Setear:

Synonym of camping, or camping, also with negative connotations.

Stomp:

From the English to stomp (to stomp very hard). Win an online game decisively.

Taunt:

From English to taunt (to mock). Make mocking movements to provoke the opponent and try to get him to make an attack movement. Very common in fighting games.

Troll:

Person who posts messages that are generally provocative or offensive in chats, forums, social networks, etc. with the sole purpose of generating controversy or disturbing the rest of the participants in the community.

Featured English-speaking video game slang terms:

1-Up:
An extra life.

Adds:
Additional monster summoned by one you are fighting.

Aggro:
When a monster is irritated and focused on you.

AFK:
Away from keyboard. Away from the keyboard.
Aimbot:
A cheat mechanism that automatically targets you.
AoE:
An area of effect attack. That is, an attack with an extension of 360 degrees.
Boa:
Bind on account. An in-game item linked to your account.
Buff/Debuff:
A buff adds powers to your character; A debuff removes powers from your character.
Camp:
Hide and wait for enemies.
CB/OB:
CB – Closed Beta, OB – Open Beta. They are both games that you can try before they are released properly.
CD:
Cooldown- The recharge time after using a special power.
DPS:
Damage per second: a calculation of how much damage per hit you generate and how fast you can attack.
Dungeon:
A closed area of a game with powerful enemies and great rewards.
EXP/XP:
Experience points- The points you earn for completing tasks to increase your character's level.
FoV:
Field of view: the range of peripheral vision on the screen.
GG:
Good game.
Glitches:
A bug in the game that can give the player an advantage.
Grind:
Complete repeated tasks to earn XP points.
H.P.:
Health/Hit Points: The measure of how much life your character has left.

HUD/UI:
*Heads-up Display / User interface:*displaying your player status, skills and spells.
KDR/KR:
*Kill-to-death ratio/kill ratio:*is the number of enemies you killed compared to the number of deaths you had.
Lag:
A network or processing delay that slows down the response time of your game.
Lot:
Items that drop from enemies or that you find while exploring.
Mod:
A mod is a modification that alters the game in some way.
PM:
*Mana/Magic points:*allows you to perform magical abilities.
Nerf:
A game update that limits the power of a powerful weapon or ability.
NPC:
A non-player character: A non-player character who often advances the game's story.
Noob/Newbie:
An inexperienced newcomer to a game.
Ping:
The measurement of time in milliseconds between the player's console/computer and the host server.
OP:
*Overpowered:*a weapon or ability that is disproportionately powerful compared to other elements of the game.
PvE:
Player vs Environment- When fighting a non-player enemy.
PvP:
*Player vs Player:*when you fight another player's character.
QTE:
*Quick Time Event:*is a video game section that requires timed button presses.
Ragequit:
When you leave a game angry after losing a match.
RAID:
Team quest, usually in a single dungeon, including important

boss encounters.
Skin:
A cosmetic change to your character's appearance.
Tag:
The online name of a player. In MMORPGs, tag also refers to
identifying a target enemy of a group.

Usually, the fears that mothers and fathers have when our children
show a lot of interest in the world of video games have to do with the
risks that actually exist. Without trying to dwell too much on them,
which are surely familiar to all of us,byOn the one hand, there is the
risk of excessive social isolation at a stage where personal interactions
are very necessary. A high interest in video games could be indicative
of difficulties when establishing personal relationships. And hiding in
them can aggravate the situation, since it is common for them to
generate a lack of interest in other social or recreational activities,
which in the end would mean lost opportunities to socialize.

On the other hand, their self-esteem may suffer from being
constantly exposed to a competitive world. Comparison to other
players can make you feel like you don't measure up if you don't meet
certain standards you've previously set for yourself. And even if he
achieves them, he is not without risk, since his self-esteem could
depend more on how he is perceived by other online players, rather
than how he values himself. Video games often offer tangible forms of
validation, such as in-game achievements or comments from other
players, designed to generate that need in the user. When they spend
hours playing video games, they aren't always having a good time.
Sometimes they are fighting for themselves. They need to do it because
they cannot look each other in the face again until they achieve their
goals. And that feeling, at an age in which every feeling is magnified,
can lead to consequences that are not at all desirable.

Furthermore, video games offer us alternative realities, parallel
universes in which the player only has to create an avatar to travel to
them. An avatar that is often an idealized representation of oneself.
The comparison with his avatar and the positive sensations he
experiences while playing can lead him to underestimate his worth in
offline situations and therefore, to progressively disconnect from
reality.

The first signs that can alert us to these risks can be found in their academic life, where difficulties usually appear. The most common have to do with concentration difficulties and poor time management. Indeed, immersion in video games and the constant viewing of vYoonline games could make it difficult for adolescents to concentrate on academic tasks, since they do not have the stimuli designed for this purpose that video games do. Study forces the student to be disciplined, while games invite you to enjoy from the first moment. Additionally, the studio does not offer the immediate rewards that video games do. Digital distractions could therefore affect your ability to study, understand concepts, and complete schoolwork. If we add to this the limited investment of time for academic tasks to the detriment of the time invested in video games, the result is lower academic performance.

Many risks to take in exchange for little, just a time of fun. In my case, as a father, the temptation to answer "no", to prohibit my son from using it, was gaining more and more strength. But there was something that didn't fit. These risks did not at all describe the profile of Sergio, a student who could be considered a model. They didn't fit Diego's way of being either. Not even with Paula who, although she needs to improve academically, enjoys (excessively) a wonderful life outside of video games. The case of Sergio, Diego, Paula and so many others, made me suspect that video games not only have negative aspects to assume in exchange exclusively for fun. Also, as we can affirm after the research that Borja and I have carried out, they can be very useful to us. They are useful, for example, to discover tastes and interests that allow them to get to know each other (and us to get to know them). Furthermore, video games are excellent enhancers of many of our children's skills and virtues, which will most likely be in high demand in the increasingly technological world in which they will become adults. They can even help them develop those skills that are less present in them, playing voluntarily or applying them in a classroom or in therapy sessions. Observing them when they play, listening to them when they speak their gamer Slang, can give us a lot of information about positive aspects of our child that allow us to get to know him beyond the image he projects as a tedious idiot, only interested in passing time. That is why we think it is important to collect here the keys that allow them to have the broadest possible vision of video games and their children.

First of all, a teenager who shows a high interest in video games, to the point of using their slang in other facets of his life, is likely to have discovered a true passion. Perhaps as an advantageous aspect, it may seem like a small thing to us, but not all advantages should be based on practicality if what we want is not only for them to be able to look for life, but to live it happily. Which of you, of us, can enjoy life without the passion with which we live what makes us happy?

Focusing on more practical aspects, we can highlight how the use of video games and the correct use of their Slang are indicative of a high capacity for technological adaptation. That is to say, the person who uses them naturally has the ability to understand and adapt quickly to the technological innovations that arise, something that we know is very necessary and increasingly in demand, especially if, as happens to me, when we finally learn to use our mobile phone, it is just when the time has come to renew it and learn to use a new one.

On the other hand, any Slang (in this case that related to video games), as an element of communication, is an indication that a social interaction is taking place. Indeed, many video games, increasingly, move away from that idea that those of a certain age still maintain, of being an isolated leisure element, tied to a machine located in the solitude of a room. Today, its design involves interaction with other players, either in online multiplayer or through in-game chats. Hence the construction of such a rich own Slang. And the design of portable or mobile gaming devices capable of playing powerful video games allows them to be enjoyed in a shared environment, also facilitating in-person socialization.

Also, as we have said, video games can be a powerful tool that allows us to enhance our children's skills. Some terms in this Slang are related to strategies and tactics that must be carried out in games. Using this type of Slang suggests that they have analytical and strategic skills, which will be very useful in various aspects throughout their lives. Other terms refer more to creative or specific aspects of a specific video game, around which a community is created. If our children use Slang of this type, they show that they feel part of a community, in which they can develop their creativity, feeling free to express themselves and share their creations.

Furthermore, in a world that evolves at breakneck speed, it is necessary for our children to develop the ability to adapt to changes. The rapid evolution of video game Slang, constantly influenced by technical updates and trends of the moment, shows that those who use it are aware of the latest developments and know how to adapt quickly to changes.

Lastly, they can be very useful to us as parents when it comes to providing professional guidance. If our children show a great passion for video games, speak their Slang, know their mechanics in depth and enjoy enhancing their skills with them, they will probably be interested in future career opportunities related to their programming or design. But not only that, video games could be the gateway to a whole world of technical careers, the so-called STEM, in which they finally develop professionally.

These are, in general terms, the main risks and the main advantages that video games entail. We have intended with this information that you can accompany your children in this world that is often new for us, parents. But no matter how much information we have, it is still very difficult to avoid the fear of deciding about what we do not know, or what we know, especially because of the risks it entails. We naturally say "no" when our daughter or our son presents us with a dilemma of this type. And this does not have to be bad, as it allows us to gain the time we need to inform ourselves and offer a more thoughtful response. However, we must be aware that we do not solve the problem if we claim it as a definitive answer, without a thoughtful argument to accompany it. With the "no", we have only kicked the ball forward. An open and unconditional "yes" is not the best idea either, no matter how many advantages video games can provide. None of us would let our children go ahead if we were exploring a forest for the first time, even if that forest ended up being beautiful. The decision is never easy and doubts always accompany. For this reason, we tend to simplify its complexity by looking for the correct answer in a figure, a specific age in our children, with which, if we manage to retain them until we reach it, we have the feeling of having done our job well. But the previous metaphor continues to serve us to question this reasoning: At what age would we let our children go alone?a strangerforest? Ten, twelve, sixteen…?

This is not a book on family communication per se, although we do seek to promote such communication by shedding light on the Slang they speak and everything it can help us get to know them. But having come this far, now in confidence, we hope you don't mind if we dare to offer you some advice: to make this type of decision, more important than when is how. There are as many types of adolescents and families as there are people in the world. It is a chimera to recommend an age on which we would all agree. However, as good mothers and fathers that we are (because if we have reached our children's adolescence, we will not be doing anything wrong), we know the importance of accompanying them in their growth. Now it shouldn't be any different. The only differenceliesin that until now we knew the terrain and felt safe guiding them, and now we have to demand that we keep up to date with a whole new world that is opening up to our children.

There is a lot of literature, a lot of information on the Internet, as well as parental control tools, that can help us configure that "how" in the way that best suits our needs, allowing us to set the conditions that we consider appropriate to allow our children move forward in these new worlds. If in this way we manage to foster a healthy balance between allowing them time online and teaching them to also enjoy the real world, inviting them to participate in activities that promote, like video games, a sense of achievement and self-esteem, such as playing a sport. , creative hobbies in which they must make something of their own, or even community activities, we can achieve it. And if we accompany this with open conversations that emphasize the importance of valuing ourselves for our character, skills and personal achievements beyond video games, we will have done a very good job. Good luck with such an exciting company! Do we dare now with social media?

3. SOCIAL MEDIA SLANG

"It does not have to be this way". Marina did not doubt that what I was saying was true, but she also did not hesitate to intervene to correct me. We had literally exchanged four words: her "thank you" in response to my "hello, good. Welcome" had been all. The new art teacher was a very young woman, about twenty-five years old, and at that moment I associated her spontaneous intervention with the arrogant impetus typical of her age. But she was wrong...

Now that we are good friends, I fondly remember that first conversation with Marina, precisely with social networks as a common thread. I had just entered the staff room. I was worried about two students from my tutoring, new to the institute because their activity on networks had generated such problems for them that they had to change centers. I felt, we feel, a lot of helplessness, since it is very difficult for teachers to prevent such conflicts that arise in the online universe. We dedicate our efforts to giving generic talks and workshops that everyone receives together, in a mass that we can hardly personalize. Of course, although these problems arise on the Internet, far from where we can prevent them, the consequences do explode with all their virulence within the walls of the school. As a tutor, one often feels like a firefighter in the middle of a fire, trying to put out the flames with hardly any resources, with blows.

Added to my concern for my students was my personal experience with social networks, which did not exactly help to see them in a better light. I wasn't born with them. Let's say, without revealing the impertinent date of my birth, that I remember watching the fall of the Berlin Wall on television. For this reason, my relationship with social networks was a posteriori, as an adult. They are useful to me to maintain contact with family and friends from a distance or to follow some accounts of people whose content I find interesting. I don't enjoy that exhibitionist aspect, in which you have to show practically at every moment where you are and what you are doing at that moment. On the other hand, the idea of exchanging opinions, of debating current affairs or more important topics was attractive to me. I express it in the past tense after having learned that this idea is far from reality, after several unpleasant encounters with other users in which insults replaced arguments. On networks like X (the old Twitter), it seems to be the main entertainment.

Why is there so much hate on networks? Shouldn't they serve to connect strangers instead of confronting them? From Psychology, some answers are offered that help explain (not understand) the tendency of a large number of social network users towards insults and disqualification. They explain, therefore, the existence of trolls, those large, rude, dangerous and silly mythological beings, who, it seems,they like to acquirea mobile phone from which to pour out his bile. And, currently, the term troll is widely used to describe people who intervene or start conversations with the aim of provoking, offending, attracting attention or boycotting a dialogue. There are several factors that Psychology highlights:

Depersonalization of the individual: By not having the other person in front of us, the ethical and moral barriers that we have in mind when we give our opinions and disagree in person are blurred, objectifying our neighbor. It also happens to us behind the wheel, where our attitudes become more aggressive when shouting at other vehicles and not so much at other people.

Feeling of anonymity: Hidden behind a nickname, some people feel less inhibited and more likely to express themselves in a brusque and disrespectful way, something they would not do in their real life. Anonymity removes ethical barriers, thus increasing aggressive behavior in a conversation.

Absence of non-verbal communication: 85% of communication is non-verbal. As it is not possible in networks, alterations occur in the transmission and clarity of messages, giving rise to misunderstandings that are the source of conflict.

De-responsibility and absence of a control group: Showing opinion in the digital sphere, together with the aforementioned anonymity, makes the feeling of responsibility for our actions less. Furthermore, by not being in a physical group context when making a comment, you avoid constant regulation and correction by the ethical and moral norms that emanate from the strength of the group.

Relativization of time/space: The Internet makes it easier to interact beyond our geographical context and time zone, allowing us to judge, in a completely decontextualized way, facts that are poorly understood in our local environment, out of context.

Bubble filter: Social networks often show us content that coincides with the beliefs and opinions that we already have and have been expressing, even if in a veiled way, through them. This creates "bubbles" in which interacting people think similarly. When this happens and our opinions are accepted and applauded, people tend to be burdened with reason and become intransigent with those who express different opinions who, in turn, are equally intransigent, generating conflict.

That the presence of trolls is so common in the digital world has to do with the simplicity that the network offers to fulfill, without much effort, our need to belong to a group (participating with the masses in discrediting to theother, in insulting the new or different...) and to enhance individual prestige (not by exalting one's own qualities, but by humiliating or mocking the opponent). Both, needs arising from life in common with others, which we tend to cover with social networks, as we will see later.

In short, we can assure that trolls exist and not only in stories. There are also them on social networks. And the frequent encounter with them is what led me to abandon some social network and my two new students, to have to change schools. Hence that day, returning to the anecdote of my first meeting with Marina, I entered the teachers' room ranting about social networks, so convinced of the evil they represent. He argued that they are a coercive instrument, that they limit the user's freedom in the worst possible way: with self-censorship. If we do not want to be insulted, disqualified, repudiated or marginalized, we have no choice but to act under the direction of political correctness, publish only what is expected of us in advance, or limit ourselves to having a more passive than active role, simply dedicating ourselves to like to attract friends who respond in a similar way.

"It doesn't have to be like that, they help me to be able to express myself freely," Marina interrupted me.

The conversations with my new partner have made me reflect a lot during this time. Because of her youth, social networks have been part of Marina's life since her adolescence, and have helped shape her adult personality. Today, if there is one word to define it, it is freedom. But there was a time when it wasn't like that. A time in which her personal relationships, in an adolescence limited to a high school, were scarce if not painful. She did not find anyone in her immediate environment with whom to share her passion, anime, and that generated a social isolation that left her.andconditioned some years. "On social media I have felt more listened to than I have felt all my life.ThereI found a way to travel far to find people like me and share a true friendship with them. I also learned to relate openly, developing an ironic vein and an unfiltered sense of humor, which I apply to my art to break down some of the walls of a social construct in which there was no space for me."

Today, Marina is an artist of some prestige. She enjoys a large online community (including myself) with whom she shares her art. She knows many of them in person, from her exhibitions or from the exhibitions of other artists that she attends. And her closest friendships emerged from those contacts through social networks. Of course she has encountered unpleasant situations, even provoking them with her art. But it's worth it to her. She prefers to enjoy the freedom of it without being conditioned by the consequences. A freedom learned in the virtual world, which she has been able to transfer to her real life. Marina lives her life freely. On the other hand, I, more restrained in my way of being, transfer my scruples to my online profile. My modesty, turned into self-censorship on social networks. Are social networks therefore the cause ofhow muchDo we dislike them, or are they simply a tool in which those things that we decide to show or hide will be reflected? I'm not clear about the answer. I leave the conclusions to this reflection to you.

If as adults we find it difficult to understand everything that social networks entail, let's imagine what they mean for a teenager. Their emotional vulnerability, in a phase of life of profound physical, emotional and identity changes; The social pressure to which they are subjected due to the need to fit in and be accepted by the group, and their immaturity when evaluating the risks of what they show or when facing the unpleasant moments they experience on social networks, make them be the perfect victims. There are many risks to which they are exposed when becoming users of a social network:

On the one hand, social networks are designed to be addictive and they manage to be so for a very high percentage of users. In Spain, for example, 50% of adolescents abuse, or do not use, their mobile phone, using it more than five hours a day, mainly on social networks. Talks to prevent addictions among young people, which previously focused on tobacco, alcohol and substances considered soft drugs, now focus on technological addictions and addictions derived from the use of technology, such as pornography or online gaming.

These additions have to do with the possibility that technology offers them to access a whole world of inappropriate content, mainly violent or sexual in nature, which also tends to be frequently shared on a social network among the members of a group, since being aware that they are accessing adult content, it is considered by young people as an element of prestige: the one who sees, knows and shares the most, the older and more worldly they are considered. We will develop the risks involved in the recurring consumption of this type of content in a teenager in a later chapter, which unfortunately is more frequent than we would like.

Social networks are also a risk element that can undermine your self-esteem. The negative social comparison that occurs between a real life and the carefully crafted lives that are shown on social networks is behind many of the psychological disorders that our adolescents suffer: depression, anxiety, the appearance of eating disorders... They are well known and admired the influencers. Even our children have been able to tell us that they want to be an influencer when they grow up. It is a necessity in adolescence to find role models that help them grow. But if there are influencers it is because there are impressionable. If the messages of those who imitate are not appropriate, there is a risk that their way of acting will have negative consequences, such as, for example, carrying out dangerous viral challenges that periodically become fashionable.

The need to capture the attention of others and the autonomy that a mobile phone offers to adolescents, which makes them have a word processor, recorder, camera, video camera and Internet connection in their pocket, make them very much victims. frequency of privacy loss. It is true that, at certain ages, it is very difficult for them to adequately evaluate the consequences of an exhibition that they consider intimate, in a global environment with no privacy. But it's not always like this. On many occasions, they are aware of the risks, but the need for acceptance from others also drives them to assume them. This entails other greater risks, such as grooming, a practice in which an adult pretends to be a minor to once gain the trust of his or her child or adolescent interlocutor, or once he or she has certain information with which to blackmail him or her, obtain images yours with high sexual content.

Either because of their own information that a teenager has posted on a social network, believing themselves to be in an environment of trust, or because other teenagers use the capacity that their mobile phone offers them to record, speak, write and publish on networks about others, one of the main risks of social networks is cyberbullying or cyberbuying. We are more sensitive to this risk than to others, since the serious consequences that bullying has on the emotional well-being of adolescents are known to all. At its highest point, suicide, which in Spain accounts for just over 30% of the deaths of adolescents between 12 and 17 years old (32.3% in the last published report). But without reaching the tip of the iceberg, there are many other serious consequences of being subjected to the constant ridicule that social networks allow, twenty-four hours a day, seven days a week, at a vital moment in which belonging to the group is essential for the development of the individual. Without going into detail, let's say that under that permanent magnifying glass emotional well-being is impossible.

As expected, one of the first consequences of inappropriate use of social networks is the impact they generate on academic performance, which plummets when the adolescent's goals move away from academic goals, or when they suffer in their academic performance. person any of the indicated risks. The positive thing about bad results appearing immediately is that they can be the alert that makes us suspect that something is starting to go wrong. It is important to be attentive to these alerts to act quickly and prevent more serious consequences. As a teacher, there are many interviews with families in which we start talking about school performance and end up detecting much more complex problems, which require the help of the school counselor or directly from an external professional.

Over the years, there are many names of students that come to mind. Many painful failures, but also many strategies that were successful. The problem is that there are no magic wands, nor certainties that guarantee that the steps taken are not taken incorrectly. What worked once, doesn't work another time. And if the certainties are scarce and the risks so serious, the doubts that we as parents may have had when allowing them to use video games, now appear again, much more pronounced if possible: Why should we consider allowing them to use social networks? The short answer is shocking: they need them. They are for them a natural way of relating and finding role models that allow them to define themselves as adults. But this would be more Marina's brusque style. We prefer to offer you a broader answer, with the aim of encouraging thoughtful and serene reflection on its use. Because, even if we are convinced of it, it is not easy to defend to people like you, who go out of their way to guarantee the safety of their children, that adolescents need such a dangerous tool. However, we are also convinced that not only do they go out of their way to guarantee the safety of their daughters and sons, but what they really would like is to guarantee their well-being. Although for this they make use of what is scary; although their decisions do not coincide with those we would make; Although their passions do not fit with ours, let us understand that they are just what makes them happy. That's why the decisions we have to make as parents are so complex. Hence, it is not easy to explain to them why they need social networks.

It is best to start at the beginning: already in ancient times, Aristotle described human beings as a social being by nature. And indeed, we need the rest of the individuals that make up our society to cover our basic needs, which is why we tend to live in it. But the mere fact of living in society generates, in turn, other types of less material needs, gestated in the psyche of every individual who lives in society, which are also magnified if that individual is an adolescent: need for approval and belonging to a group, and need for personal prestige.

The first, the need for approval and belonging to a group, is characterized by the search for one or several specific social groups (family, religion, etc.).territory, gender, culture, age, etc.) with which to identify. This identification forces individual behaviors to be modeled to a large extent to facilitate acceptance, cohesion and coexistence with the rest of the group, thus avoiding their rejection. If a Muslim or a Christian has to go to their mosque or church to meet the group and celebrate their ritual together, a teenager, who due to age has limited movement on the physical level, finds his temple on the social network, and It will modulate its behaviors to adapt them to that environment.

Furthermore, living in society provokes in the individual the need for prestige within his or her reference group, in which, by bringing out his or her strengths, he or she tries to climb the ladder or become significant to the rest. That is why it is so important for a teenager to publish content about himself and his strengths, and he is so in need of likes that make him see that he is important to the group.

To meet these needs, social networks offer many advantages. As we have already seen, it is easy to cover both by becoming a troll, but, although they are a dangerous tool when used incorrectly, they are a very useful tool in adolescence, where they have become the main instrument for socializing.

This would be the first and fundamental advantage: social networks are one of the main means of social contact. They allow them to stay in touch with friends and classmates, as well as make new friends, even if there are enormous distances between them. This is especially important at a stage of life in which social relationships are fundamental and in which contacts on the physical level are very limited by age, since they are reduced to a certain distance from the home and certain schedules that are considered appropriate.

In line with the above, as happened to Marina, social networks can help adolescents develop their social skills. For many, the distance that occurs in online contact is the security cover they lack in person. And wrapped in that covering, they dare to get rid of their shell and learn to communicate with the other, to know them and to make themselves known.

Precisely to make themselves known, social networks are an excellent platform, allowing them to express their identity, their interests and their personality through photos, publications and status updates.

And through these manifestations, adolescents can find the perfect space to explore their identity and learn to know themselves. In them they can explore, with a certain intimacy regarding their family environment, different aspects of their identity, such as their sexual orientation, their gender identity or the personal beliefs that will make up their ideology. They are the ideal space to meet new references, who show different aspects from those instilled in the family and school environment. Although we have already seen that there are negative ones, on social networks there are also positive models to imitate, which help them grow. Important people in their lives that, if it weren't for the social network, it would have been impossible for them to meet.

Of course, social networks also offer much more practical advantages, as an entertainment tool, a learning tool or an active information channel, with the possibility not onlyforknow about something, but to mobilize about it, as is the case with youth mobilizations against climate change.

At this point, if we understand that they are as dangerous as they are at the same time so positive, we may be considering their use. The question then should be how do we do it? Answering these questions would be much easier if we didn't love them so much. We would have many fewer doubts and we could be much more decisive to finally live in peace. But we can't help loving them, just as we can't avoid risks. What we can do is prevent and minimize them. We have to accompany our daughter or our son in this world, as we already did with video games. Of course, on this occasion, we must keep in mind that we must do it at an age in which the advantages offered by social networks are beneficial for them. Unlike video games, the how and when are equally important here. There are video games adapted to all ages, but they do not exist, they do not need, social networks before social relationships are a fundamental part of their lives. Usually, the minimum age to have social networks is fourteen years old, but the mechanisms to control age when registering on any social network are minimal. It is very easy for our teenagers to create an account at a younger age, or we may have even thought it appropriate to allow it as an element of entertainment. But we must be aware that the usefulness of a social network in childhood is reduced to mere entertainment. The risks, however, are the same, if possible accentuated by the infant's lower maturity.

Once the when has been established, to help us define how, we suggest applying the same guidelines that we recommend when deciding on the use of video games: we must be informed of everything that concerns social networks to try to stay one step ahead of them. our daughters and sons and thus be able to guide them properly; We have to know the tools that allow us to carry out parental control that gives them the autonomy they need, and gives us the security we need. And we have to talk a lot with them, reinforce their self-esteem, help them.eitherknow how to make mature decisions, assessing the consequences, to be resilient...

Talking a lot with them is easy to say or write in this case, but that communication is neither as easy nor as fluid as we would like. Let's not forget that we have before us a teenager, whose speech is built on the basis of monosyllables, acronyms and encrypted expressions that could perfectly well be used in the invocation of some demon. That is why it is so important to understand them, to be able to accompany them properly, to know their Slang. On social networks especially. It is your main means of communication. Knowing what they say, we will know how they are, how they feel and if we need to be vigilant against any of the risks described. And if we have this invaluable information, our communication with them will be more meaningful. We will be able to adequately focus our mother or father lessons on their demands, making it easier for our messages to penetrate.

We have selected some of the main terms used in both Spanish and English-speaking slang. However, it is very common for acronyms and abbreviations to be used on social networks, used in a similar way regardless of the cultural context in which they are developed. Their use is so popular because it is an agile and quick way to express oneself, but also because the message you want to express can be hidden in them, so it is important to know them to prevent some of the risks they entail. Although we will develop this in a later chapter, as an example, the acronyms THOT, HOE, BOSH SBW or SLUB are useful, all of them with the same and derogatory meaning (whore).

Acronyms and abbreviations most used in social networks:

+1:
It is equivalent to "like". That is, it serves to recommend content or recognize your interest.
AFAIK(As far as I know):
AFAIK; as far as I understand
AFK(Away From Keyboard):
It is used to indicate that you will be away from the keyboard or "Not Available", in the middle of a video game or chat conversation.
ASAP(as soon as possible):
Translate "as soon as possible." It can be used in conversations like "I need that information asap."
B.N.:
The abbreviation of "Good."
BRB (Be right back):
I'll be right back.
BTW (By the way):
By the way.
DIY(do it yourself):
Translates "do it yourself." It is seen more on YouTube and Facebook.
DM(direct message):
Direct message. It is used in X (Twitter).
Fail and Win:
Translated it would be "Failure and Success". It is used to express emotion or mockery at the failure of another.
FIY(For your information):
For your information; so you know.
FOMO (fear of missing out):
Fear of missing out.

G2G (Get to go):
I have to go.
GOAT:
The acronym stands for "Greatest of All Time," which is used to refer to someone who is the best at what they do, whether in sports, music, or another area.
HTH(Hope that helps):
It is used when you share useful information with another person and say "I hope it helps you."
IDK(I don't know):
It is used to express ignorance about something.
ILY and ILU(I Love You) and (I Love U):
It is short for writing "I love you."
IMO(In my opinion):
In my opinion.
IRL(In real life):
With this acronym it is expressed that what is being told is not an invention.
JK (Just kidding):
It refers to the fact that what was just said is "just a joke."
K or KK(OK):
Okay; OK
LMK (Let me know):
Let me know.
LOL and LOLZ (Laughing Out Loud):
It is used to express laughter out loud, to point out that something is very funny.
LYKYK(if you know, you know):
You know what I mean.
MOOD:
It refers to the mood to do some activity. It is seen in expressions like "I'm not in the mood."
OMG(Oh my God or oh my gosh):
It is used to express amazement.
ROFL(rolling on the floor):
Hilarious.
RT(Retweet):
Forward a message on X (Twitter).
TBH (To be honest):
Sincerely; in fact.

TBT(throwback Thursday):
"Memory of the past". It is used to remember an old publication or photo.
THX (Thanks):
"Thank you". A quick thank you.
TL;DR(too long; didn't read):
Too long, I haven't read it.
X2:
It is used to express that you agree with a comment said previously. If someone else has already used it, you can say "X3", "X4", etc.
YOLO (you only live once):
You only live once.

Most common terms of social media slang in Spanish:

01, 02, 05…:
It is the way that young people indicate their year of birth and therefore, refer to their age. For example, 01 would be 2001.
Aesthetic:
This term can be translated as visually attractive. It is used to define a type of aesthetic that always seeks to exalt beauty, regardless of the field.
Beef:
Originally, this word was only used in the world of hip hop or trap. Nowadays, its use has extended to everyday speech and refers to the hints that two or more individuals give to each other in a confrontational tone. It can also be used when the fight is physical.
Binge:
Also known as "binge-watch". Habit of binge-watching multiple episodes of a television series online.
Boomer:
Technically, they are those people who were born between 1946 and 1964. However, members of Generation Z use it to refer to those people who do not understand their codes.
Boque:
The expression being a "boque" or "un boquerón" is a colloquial expression used by Generation Z, which refers to a person who has never kissed someone. It has a derogatory

connotation that describes a person's lack of experience in romantic relationships.

Bro:
Abbreviation of "brother". It is one of the terms that young people use to refer to their friends or colleagues.

Cayetano:
Term popularized on social networks to refer to what was previously called 'posh', that is, young people from a wealthy social class who like to be dressed in clothes from famous brands and at high prices.

Cringe:
Cringe is an Anglo-Saxon term that has become popular worldwide thanks to the internet and social networks. It is used to describe a reaction of embarrassment or discomfort in a specific situation or behavior. Alludes to moments that are embarrassing or difficult to watch.

Crush:
Translated from English, it can mean "to crush", "to fail" or "to crush", but in the language of love it adopts another definition: "platonic love" or "crush". This meaning is the most used in social networks. Therefore, a crush is called a sudden infatuation that is deeply passionate, reveals, excites and excites, regardless of whether it is feasible or not, as if it were a spell.

De Chill:
The word 'chill' comes from English and translated into Spanish means "cool". It also refers to relaxing or something being "relaxed" or "calm." The term has actually been used for a long time among gamers, to make their teammates understand not to move so fast or to calm down their actions within the game. In addition, "chill" has been part of other popular phrases, such as the famous expression "Netflix and chill", which is used on social networks to indirectly talk about a sexual encounter. Now, apart from all its previous uses, the word "chill" is once again used as a synonym for a joke when users say "it's from chill" or "from chill." In this way they make the other person understand that they should not take what happened personally, because it is just a joke and they should not get angry. It is usually accompanied by the emoji of the little hand with a surfer pose, a hand that has only the

thumb and little finger extended.

De locos:
Way of indicating that what is being talked about seems fantastic to you, you love it.

El Alucin:
El Alucin is a term that refers to the altered state of consciousness caused by drugs. However, among young people it is used to describe someone who likes to appear to have a lot and show off more than they really have. It is now beginning to be used in a broader sense, to describe any person who usually tells a notable number of lies.

Fachero:
Person of good taste, who cares a lot about grooming and dress. It can also refer to an object or situation to indicate that something is attractive or fun.

Flamer:
Term used to describe the person who is dedicated to insulting and creating controversy with the aim of igniting a conversation. Similar, therefore, to troll.

Ghosting:
The expression "ghosting" someone is used when a relationship with another person, whether romantic or friendship, is suddenly broken. There are different types of ghosting, but, in general, the person who "ghosts" another person decides to stop communicating with them from one day to the next.

Hype:
Get overly excited about something. It is also used to describe something or someone that is in fashion, although it is expected to be temporary.

Lache:
Synonym of "cringe", that is, embarrassment of others. Although it can also be translated as disgust or even laziness, depending on the context.

The 'jennys':
Way of referring to girls who, like the MDLR, like to dress in tracksuits and other sports clothing, accompanied by non-sporty accessories such as large hoop earrings, rings, etc. Before, the term 'choni' was used more, but as has happened with 'posh', it has been replaced among the new generations

by 'jennys'.
Lit:
It is the abbreviation of "literally" or "literally", used to highlight the literal meaning of what is said or to make the interlocutor see that you agree with what is said. It can also be an expression used to express that something has a value. very positive for the speaker, that is, as a synonym for "great" or "excellent."
MDLR:
It is the abbreviation of Mec de la rue, a French term whose translation would be "street boy." It has been made popular among young people, in part, by singer Morad, a 23-year-old artist born in Spain and of Moroccan descent who describes himself on his Instagram account as "MDLR Ni madero ni chivato." In his songs, he talks about what life is like in a working-class neighborhood, loyalty between friends or the difficulties of getting ahead. This term is used among young people to refer to boys from working-class families who have been on the streets since they were very young, looking for a life for themselves and their family. Sometimes it is used in a derogatory way, to criticize an aesthetic considered 'cani', characterized by usually dressing in tracksuits or sports clothing and non-sports accessories, such as chains, rings or bracelets. Other times, MDLR is used as a way to express the fight against any type of social discrimination.
NPC:
NPC stands for Non Playable Character. Although its origin is found in video games, it is commonly used on social networks to talk about people without their own opinions, who do not think for themselves or who behave in a predictable way. It can also be used, although to a lesser extent, to refer to people who are in the background, not very relevant in the life of the person making the mention.
NTR:
Acronyms for "don't even scratch yourself". Used to express that there is no need to worry or give too much importance to something in particular.
Panas:
Group of friends.

Padrear:

Padrear is used when a person says or does something that provokes tremendous admiration at a certain moment among his audience. It can be used in the first person when one wants to show off or act cool. Now, those attitudes are called "parenting."

Periodt:

It is used to settle a phrase that one believes can hardly be refuted. Its origin comes from the word "period" (period, in Spanish). Some users indicate that, with the 't' added at the end, the aim is to place more emphasis on the pronunciation.

Picket:

If for the Royal Spanish Academy, a picket is a wound made with a sharp instrument or a group of people trying to impose or maintain a strike slogan, for young people this word is also synonymous with 'flow', that is, style. innate. You can say, for example, "The clothes are bought, but the picket is not."

POV:

POV is the English acronym for point of view. It comes from cinema and is commonly used on social networks. It is used to show the way we react that we have or would have when something happens to us, telling it, therefore, from a personal point of view.

Random:

This word can be translated from English as "random" and used to refer to something coincidental, that has not been planned. It can also be used when something is strange, which generates strangeness.

Ratio:

It is used to express disagreement with a comment made on networks, usually on X (Twitter). Many users respond directly to a publication by putting a "ratio" to express that they do not like anything and disagree or suggest others "ratio" certain messages.

Red Flag:

A "red flag" is a warning or alarm regarding a type of attitude or behavior that is not appropriate for a person, such as jokes that border on disrespect or attitudes that are not appropriate to the context.

Roast:
Informal English expression that means "to make fun of." Making a roast on YouTube consists of making a video reviewing some of the insulting comments that your haters make to you.

Salseo:
Any controversy or controversy carried out on social networks that users like to comment on.

Ship:
It translates as the desire or preference for two people, generally fictional characters, to have a relationship. The expression derives from the English word "relationship" (relationship in Spanish), from which came "to ship", which is to ship in the naturalized version in our language. From this term are derived the "ship names", that is, the new name created by the fans of two famous people, to refer to them as a couple. For example, Brangelina to refer to the couple formed by the actors Brad Pitt and Angelina Jolie. .

Si soy:
It is an expression used to indicate that one feels identified with a publication or a situation. Thus, simply, it is the response given after the situation raised by the interlocutor.

Stalking:
It comes from the English word stalk and means gossiping about the profiles of other users on social networks, whether famous people or anonymous people who have piqued your interest.

You need a street:
An older expression, but very popular on social networks. It is used to indicate that someone has little experience in something or that they simply lack experience.

Trend:
It is the way of expressing that something is trending. Tik Tok virals are also called that.

Twinning:
It comes from the English term "twin", which means "twin" and in social networks it is understood as dressing the same as another person. Until now, that had negative connotations, as it was an embarrassing situation. However, it is something that is now celebrated and even provoked by being fashionable.

Vibes:

The word "vibes" refers to the sensations that a situation, a context, a place or a person gives off in the subject. It can be with positive or negative connotations, talking about good vibes or bad vibes.

Featured English-speaking social media slang terms:

Bae:

An affectionate way to refer to your partner, close friend or someone special in your life. It comes from "before anyone else."

BASIC:

This adjective is used as a kind of insult to refer to something or someone that is boring or not cool.

Boujee:

This is an adjective with which we describe something that seems luxurious, expensive or sophisticated.

Bro:

It is the abbreviation of brother and is used between friends, usually men. It's like saying "uncle" or "colleague."

Bussin:

This other adjective means "very good", "incredible" and is normally used with food, as in the following recipe titled bussing.

Chill/chill out:

This verb means relax, calm down, rest.

Cray / cray cray:

This shortened version of "crazy" means something that is out of control or something that has gotten out of someone's head.

Delulu:

It is an abbreviation of delusional which means illusory. The term originated in the K-Pop fan community to refer to the behavior of fans who create fantasies or believe that they will end up dating their idols. It is now used to describe any form of delusion.

Drip:

This adjective is also used to describe clothing or a sophisticated and modern look. TikTok users upload videos showing their "outfits" and often use this word in the titles.

Epic:

With this adjective we describe something that seems incredible, wonderful or a fantasy to us.

Was:

This term became popular on TikTok where it is used both humorously and seriously. For example, if you are in that phase of improving as a person, of taking care of yourself, of thinking about yourself, you are in your "healing era."

Extra:

It is another adjective that translates as dramatic or likes to attract attention.

Facts:

When someone says "facts", they mean that the information is a fact, a reality and the opposite cannot be denied.

Flex:

When someone "flexes," they are proudly displaying their accomplishments, skills, or possessions. It could be sharing a photo of a new car or talking about an academic achievement.

For real:

With this phrase we ask the other person if they mean what they just said.

Gatekeep:

In this internet age we live in, sharing is cooleitherAnd whoever does not do it will be said to be doing "gatekeep". That is, it refers to those people who do not share information, such as where they bought a t-shirt or where they took that cool photo.

Give the ick:

This phrase refers to a sudden feeling of disgust or repulsion towards a person, whether because of the way they dress, how they smell, or how they treat a waiter.

Glow up:

Referring to a positive transformation from the past to the present. It may be a change in appearance, confidence or personality.

I can't even:

It is a way of saying "I was speechless" and is used when something is so incredible that you have no words to describe it or also when something surpasses you.

It's giving:
This expression is used to describe that something or someone gives you good vibes. It is usually used to praise or highlight something.

Just sayin':
This expression is put at the end of sentences to show that what you just said is not what you think. Sometimes just sayin' serves to soften a sentence with bad intentions.

Legit:
Something "legit" means that something is very good. It is short for legitimate, which means authentic or real.

Lit:
This adjective is used to describe a fun situation, full of energy or also to talk about someone who is drunk.

Mag:
It is simply the abbreviation of "magazine" (magazine).

On fleek:
When something is "on fleek", it means that it is perfect or impeccable. It is often used to describe well-groomed eyebrows or well-applied makeup.

Periodt:
And period! There's nothing more to speak of!

Private not secret:
This term refers to couple photos in which one of the parties exposes the relationship, but in a somewhat private way. For example, a photo of your hands clasped or hiding the other person's face. That is, they keep their relationship private, but not secret.

Rent-free:
With this adverb we indicate that something has become an obsession, that we can't stop thinking about it.

Rizz   :
This term is often used as a shortened version of the word charisma. When someone has "rizz", it means that someone is seductive, has self-confidence, has something that makes him attractive.

Salty:
This other adverb means to exaggerate or react disproportionately to something.

Status:
It is being in that intermediate zone in which one does not know how to define a relationship well, which rotates between friendship and courtship.

Sksksk:
This expression is an onomatopoeia used to represent laughter, often in situations that are funny or adorable. It is sometimes combined with "and I oop", which comes from a viral video where someone interrupts themselves while speaking.

Slay:
It is usually used to express admiration or praise. It is widely used to describe someone or something that is very good, impressive, or distinguished.

Sliving:
This term devised by Paris Hilton means living your best life. It is the combination of two words: slay (which would be translated as "hit it" or "make it great") and living.

Squad:
Your "squad" is your close group of friends with whom you spend a lot of time and share experiences.

Their:
The abbreviation for "suspicious". That is, something or someone is suspicious.

Torch:
In the context of teen slang, "tea" refers to gossip or interesting, current information about people's lives. If someone says "spill the tea," it means they want you to tell them the gossip.

Thank you, next:
This colloquial term was popularized by the singer Ariana Grande and her song titled in the same way. It means "thank you, next" and means that something or someone was useful, but not anymore.

To ghost someone:
In Spanish we say "ghosting", which is basically stopping answering someone's messages or calls without giving explanations.

Totes:
Abbreviation of "totally", which is used to agree with someone

or agree with them.

Touch Grass:

This is a synonym for the phrase "get a grip!" (perhaps already a little old-fashioned for new generations), which means "calm down" or "calm down."

Vanilla:

This adjective describes something that is mediocre, boring or bland. It arises from vanilla ice cream, which is seen as a very average flavor.

Vibe check:

This term means to check if someone, spontaneously, plays along with you.

YAAASSSSSS :

It does not have a defined number of A or S and is another way of saying yes, but with a lot of enthusiasm.

As you see, they are capable of saying a lot with very little. Have they impoverished the language or have they enriched it with a multitude of nuances? This debate takes on greater significance when, to communicate, they accompany or directly replace their messages with images of all kinds: emojis, stickers, memes... Why do they use them so frequently? Do they mean the same thing as they do to us or do they use them with other meanings? Do they say a lot about our daughters and sons or are they just indicative of a lack of maturity? Should we allow their use or should we teach them to express themselves correctly?

Teenage slang, without all these graphic elements, would not be what it is today. After a chapter as complicated as this one, it doesn't hurt to let ourselves go a little and delve into this fun world. Go for it!

4. VISUAL SLANG

Dear reader: Hello.

If my greeting seemed excessively brief and even a bit abrupt or dry, we have good news for you: we don't know what your identity card reveals, but you still maintain a young spirit. If, on the other hand, I have seemed correct to them, I am afraid that they reveal that they have abandoned the youth club (twenty-somethings, thirty-somethings...) and have joined, as is my case, the even more select mature club (forty-somethings, fifties...).

I would never have believed that, by simply saying hello, I could show myself as someone stern and difficult to deal with. I thought that would happen to someone who doesn't say hello, in any case. But since the pandemic, when contact with my students began to occur not only in the classroom, but also through a virtual classroom, there were reactions of surprise when, apart from the general messages, I wrote a comment. individually to the students he knew who were going through a difficult time: "Hey, teacher, thank you very much. I didn't know you were so nice," Fran told me one day. "Thank you, teacher. You are the best. Although you seem very serious, deep down you can see that you have a big heart," he wanted to dedicate another day to me.Alexandra.

At first it was difficult for me to accept these praises full of veiled criticism. I had always considered myself an accessible teacher, who enjoyed the sympathy of his students, but overnight, that had disappeared without me having done anything to deserve it. At that moment, it was clear to me that a smear campaign was underway against me. It could not be anything else! All that was left was to know who was behind it, who was dedicated to describing me as a serious, haughty and rude person. Shortly after I understood: that person was me.

The messages he published in the virtual classroom were messages typical of a professional relationship: a generic greeting, a detailed task, and a simple farewell. Although in a context as complex as the pandemic, I was terribly concerned about the well-being of my students and tried to follow up on time in those cases in which the circumstances were especially difficult, I did not realize the importance of certain visual elements. of the language of the Internet, which incorporate into the messages received through a screen what we lack in the non-verbal communication that is established in person, and how relevant it is to understand the correct meaning of the words. As my students taught me in a reverse online class, in which I was the one taking notes of all their lessons, if I wanted to be close and convey my sincere love and concern for them, I just had to add a random number and ridiculous vowels to my generic greeting, something like "hellooooo" or in its most sweetened version, as Silvia always dedicated to me before raising a question: "hiiiiiiii." Even Eduardo, always sparse in words, was much more empathetic than me without using a single letter, simply greeting with a 👋. In that class, they talked to me about emojis and explained to me the meaning of many of them, which in some cases was different from what I gave them. They also told me about memes, touches of graphic humor that sometimes become little gems of wit. And they also taught me the importance of stickers, which are meant to be used like emojis, but they have a personal touch that says a lot about the person who uses them. After that class, our research has also led us to learn about many other forms of visual communication, such as kaomojis, sequences of characters that together form faces, gestures and emotions (less and less used); bitmojis, which are customizable avatars that are created to present ourselves online; the reactions, which are images with which we can respond (react) to the message that has reached us; or GIFs, which are animated images made from the union of several images into one, which are played as a video in a loop. But what I learned most in that class was the importance of these elements in the daily communication of adolescents and the importance, therefore, of knowing them in order to understand their messages and to be able to communicate with them, also adequately understanding our own. .

To be honest, we have doubts about giving the relevance of Slang to these visual elements, because as a backdrop, there is an open debate about whether or not their use is appropriate. Many consider them elements that impoverish communication, since they provide nuances to the conversation that could be achieved by knowing in depth the richness of the vocabulary and the strength of certain symbolic constructions, such as those of poetry. Others, however, consider them to be enriching elements, the result of the evolution of language that emerged in a digital age that has transformed our lifestyle and, therefore, our way of communicating. In fact, emojis have been recognized as relevant elements of communication even by prestigious linguistic institutions. In English, the Oxford dictionary stands out, which to date has twice chosen an emoji as 'Word of the Year' (the first time in 2015 with the emoji (face with tears of joy)). The same happens with the main institutions in Spain: the Fundéu generally declared emojis, also 'Word of the year' in 2019; and the latest edition of the dictionary of the Royal Academy of the Spanish Language (RAE) includes among its new features, the word emoji.

Without going into assessing the different points of view, what we are clear about is that young people, above all, although not exclusively, have chosen real-time communication through a screen as their main mode of interaction with others. But let us remember that 85% of communication comes from non-verbal elements, such as gestures, signals, intonations, combinations of all of them... If these elements are so relevant when it comes to properly transmitting messages, it is a logical consequence that the communication of The digital era is nourished by visual elements that seek to reproduce the context in which in-person communication occurs.

Of all the possible elements, which cannot be covered in a single chapter due to their size and the speed with which they evolve and new ones emerge, we have decided to focus on getting to know the language of emojis in more depth, as it is the most widespread element, and the of memes, as it is perhaps the one that best reflects the universality of language, being understood in a similar way regardless of the cultural context in which it occurs.

Emoji

An emoji is a small digital image or icon, 12 x 12 pixels, used in electronic communications to represent an emotion, an object, a place or an idea. Its origin dates back to 1999, when the Japanese Shigetaka Kurita created the first 176 emojis at the request of the company NTT Docomo. Today, the Unicode Consortium, the non-profit organization that is in charge of standardizing letters and characters following the Unicode system, is the one that has an Emoji Subcommittee, which is in charge of defining in this case how the most important concepts are represented. relevant globally and is concerned that they are accessible, inclusive and adequately reflect current events. At this moment, there are approximately three thousand emojis that represent emotions, natural phenomena, flags and people in various stages of life. Every day, more than seven hundred million of them are used on Facebook alone and more than half of the posts on Instagram include these elements.

If they are an element of such magnitude and so much use, it is because they are capable of fulfilling two relevant social functions. On the one hand, emojis have become a language that crosses language barriers, a universal language thanks to the fact that their visual meaning is easily understandable, regardless of the cultural context in which we find ourselves. A heart, smile, or tear emoji evokes the same feeling regardless of whether it is written in English, Spanish, or any other language. But, on the other hand, they are elements that allow messages to be transmitted that can only be understood within a community, such as a group of adolescents. Just as some emojis offer cultural nuances (such as "hands together," which can be interpreted as a prayer or expression of gratitude in some cultures, while in others it can simply represent a greeting), the perception and use of Emojis vary depending on the generation that uses them. For those of us who have seen a few primroses bloom, we tend to use emojis as an addition to the written message, fun in most uses, but not always necessary. We prefer (although the trend is changing), communication that focuses on the content of the message rather than its visual presentation. However, for younger generations, emojis are used directly as a main element in communication. With them they transmit emotions, express their identity and establish their ties of belonging to an online community. That is why we believe it is important to focus on explaining the most used emojis and especially those whose meaning varies depending on whether we or our teenage sons and daughters use them:

😂 Face crying with laughter:
It is one of the most used emojis and with a more universal meaning. It is used to denote appreciation for the humor that is developing in a relaxed context or in a comic situation, or to indicate that what one says must be taken with humor.

♡ Red heart:
Express love, affection and gratitude towards friends, family or partners. It is also used to show support or admiration for something or someone. The youngest people use it more frequently and naturally, because they do not give it the relevance that we adults give to every emotion that we dare to share. It is more difficult for us to do so, although emojis are a catchphrase that we increasingly use to communicate with the naturalness of the youngest.

😍 Face with hearts in eyes:
Here the opposite happens: while for adults it has a less profound meaning and we use it to express admiration or charm towards someone or something, for adolescents it can also indicate a strong attraction or infatuation towards a person, even if it is platonic love such as the one you have towards a celebrity.

😊 Smiling face with smiling eyes:
Another of the most used emojis and with a more universal meaning. It transmits joy, happiness and kindness and therefore, it is used to express positive emotions and to greet friends and family by sending them good wishes.

🤔 Thoughtful face:
Curiously, we use this emoji differently as adults and teenagers. We tend to use it in serious conversations or decision-making, to indicate reflection or show consideration for the important matter at hand.

However, young people use it more to show doubt or uncertainty, something like "I don't know what to do."

😢 Sad face with tears:
Universally, it is the most used emoji to express sadness or compassion for someone, especially in situations of grief or loss.

🎉 Party hat:
It is used to celebrate special occasions, achievements or moments of happiness shared with friends and followers, something we share widely.

👍 Thumbs up:
Another that is used massively and with a universal meaning: indicating approval, agreement or support for a previously expressed idea or comment.

😎 Face with sunglasses:
Much more used by teenagers than by their parents. But it is used to show that you are proud or satisfied with what you have achieved. Also to describe some situations in which you are more relaxed, such as when on vacation.

🤡 Clown:
This is an emoji used almost exclusively by young people and adolescents. It is used to represent extravagant and exaggerated humor, usually in a comedic or entertainment context. It can also be used ironically to refer to someone who is acting ridiculous or unserious, but without the negative connotations that we adults would give when using it.

💀 Skull:
Another of the emojis that adults do not use, unless we want to threaten someone with death. However, for teenagers, its meaning is very different: they use it in the same way as the acronyms LOL (Laughing Out Loud) and LMAO (Laughing My Ass Off) to indicate that they are dying of laughter.

Eggplant, fruits and other anatomical metaphors:

The eggplant has become almost universally a symbol with suggestive sexual connotations in the language of the internet and social networks. It is often used in humorous contexts or to make insinuations without having to describe the intentions, in which this vegetable represents the penis. Among adults it is used much less and if it is, it tends to be done in informal and humorous contexts.

Other images of fruits are also present in adolescent codes to refer to any part of the human anatomy that has sexual connotations. When they send the pair of cherries, refer to female breasts. And, although the use of the peach was quite widespread to refer to the ass (usually also the female one), now teenagers prefer to use the cake emoji. Even if in a derogatory way, they want to indicate that the person being talked about has a flat ass, the plate of pancakes It is his way of representing it. However, if what they want to highlight is that the person is attractive and has a good physique, they usually use the hourglass. because of the curves, it is assumed.

Brain and Peanut:

Although they do not hide any mystery for adults, young people also use them with sexual connotations. Brain is used to refer to oral sex, while peanut describes ejaculation. Both arise from wordplay associations that come from English.

Fire:

Adolescents use it to express an intense emotion but not necessarily with sexual connotations. It can reflect the enthusiasm we feel in a situation that we love or to show admiration for something exceptional done by others. Among adults it is not usually used, except in suggestive contexts, as a synonym for burning passion, although it is increasingly seen with the symbolism with which adolescents use it.

Handshake:

This emoji is used as a greeting, a sign of respect or friendship, but in a respectful way or in more formal contexts. Among adults it is used in a similar way, but we add more meanings in the professional field, where it is used to symbolize an agreement or a successful negotiation.

⭐ Star:

An emoji widely used by teenagers to decorate a message that expresses a positive emotion, happiness or admiration towards something or someone. It can also accompany messages that talk about achievements or notable moments. We adults use it much less, since we do not have as much need to accompany our messages with emojis that give emphasis to what has already been expressed.

🌈 Rainbow:

It is used with two different meanings. On the one hand, it is also used as decoration, to emphasize messages of joy or hope. On the other hand, it is used in a protesting way to defend diversity, inclusion or support for the LGBTQ+ community, whose distinctive flag is made up of the colors of the rainbow.

🤩 Face with stars in its eyes:

Generally speaking, it is an emoji that is used to convey admiration and enthusiasm for something surprising or impressive. It seeks to emphasize the intensity of the emotion.

🥰 Face with hearts:

For both the youngest and their parents, this emoji reflects love. However, while for us it is limited to expressing affection or affection for our loved ones or close friends, for teenagers it indicates falling in love. They tend to use it in love messages or romantic expressions.

🎶 Musical notes:

Widely used by teenagers as an element that accompanies and decorates any message that has to do with music: a good song that is being heard at that moment, a concert that they are going to go to or a video in which an instrument is being played. musical. As it has a decorative and emphatic use, adults again use it much less.

🍕 Pizza:

For adults, a slice of pizza is used to indicate that you eat pizza, logically. However, teenagers use it to talk about food in general. How would they feed if theyit depended? 🤤

🚀 Rocket:

The rocket emoji is used to represent excitement and enthusiasm for significant achievements. Adults also use it with this meaning, mainly in work contexts, in messages in which we want to announce the launch of a product, the launch of a project or the achievements achieved, both personal and those achieved by a work team.

🐾 Paw prints:

Another of the most used emojis to decorate messages related to pets or animals in general. Therefore, much less used by adults. However, it is also used to express the idea of following someone you admire or that someone has left a lasting mark on us.

🌊 Wave:

For adults, it symbolizes the sea, the beach or at most, using a synecdoche, vacations. However, teenagers use it mainly to greet or welcome, as if it were "hello" or rather, "helloaaaaaa".

🎭 Theatrical masks:

Although adults give it only a limited meaning, linked to the world of theater and therefore, we do not use it much, adolescents use it to point out someone who is hiding their true emotions and intentions or pretends to have a different personality.

🌻 Sunflower:

It can symbolize happiness or enjoyment of nature, but it is more common for teenagers to use it to emphasize messages of joy and positivity. Like all emojis used to decorate messages, adults use them much less.

📚 Books:

Universally, it is the emoji most used by young people and adults to refer to study and academic activities or the love of reading in general.

🎨 Color palette:

This other, on the other hand, is used by adolescents as a metaphor for having an open mind or being willing to explore new ideas. Adults use it in its strict sense, to refer to art or creativity in general.

🚲 Bicycle:

Although adults and adolescents use it to refer to outdoor activities, mainly cycling, young people also give it a connotation of freedom. They use it, therefore, to symbolize the idea of feeling free at that moment.

☕ Cup of coffee:

Like the previous one, this emoji is preferred to symbolically reflect relaxing situations in which you enjoy time at home drinking something hot. Of course, in this case, this symbolism is shared between adults and adolescents.

🏆 Trophy:

The emoji with universal meaning, mostly used to represent achievements, successes or victories. Adults, however, tend to reserve it for sporting successes.

🌙 Crescent moon:

Adults understand iteitherI consider it a reference for the night, so we use it very little. However, adolescents give it connotations of new beginnings or positive changes, thus extending its use.

👁️ 👄 👁️ Eye, lips, eye

It is a combination of emojis that teenagers use to show surprise. The surprised face 😳 It has been left for boomers like us.

This is just a selection of some of the most used emojis today, in which we have tried to represent both those used with a universal meaning, regardless of age or the cultural environment in which it occurs, as well as those that hide symbolism. used exclusively by teenagers. Of course, just as kaomojis are falling out of use, stickers are taking over emojis very quickly among the younger generations. It would not be ruled out that adults, who are having a hard time accepting emojis as another element of communication, end up using them naturally when our teenagers have found new ways to transmit their messages, ways that once again seem just as opaque as the current ones. But that is precisely the function of Slang. And that, the eternal generational struggle, in which we have the odds to lose.

However, rest assured, time is on our side. We will take revenge on them in the form of our grandchildren, when our daughters and sons have to go through the same thing they put us through, and like us, they have to succumb in the eternal generational struggle. In the meantime, let's enjoy one of the most widespread, fun and ingenious elements of Internet culture: memes. Maybe we can dedicate some of them to those teenagers who sleep under our roof. We will not win the war, but we must always give them battle.

Memes

According to the Royal Academy of the Spanish Language (RAE), which, as with the word emoji, also includes this term, a meme is an "image, video or text, usually distorted for cartoonish purposes, that is spread mainly through Internet". The word meme was coined by evolutionary biologist Richard Dawkings in his 1976 book "The Selfish Gene." In it, he uses this word as a derivative of the Greek "mimema" which refers to what is imitated, that is, what spreads from person to person. To that which, therefore, goes viral. And that is what characterizes memes, their ability to spread and spread their humor throughout the world, becoming a global phenomenon. But they are notolor humorous pieces that reach millions of people through social networks. They are also a representative part, a detailed x-ray, of the society of the moment. In a humorous way, yes, but as valuable for understanding a time as we have traditionally considered comic strips from the written press, which have been with us for several centuries and are analyzed in class as a historical document.

Memes, therefore, are not going to inform us of hidden content in the messages of our daughters and sons. Its simplicity speaks for itself, since its use is limited to generating and sharing a fun moment between the interlocutors. But they are going to give us very detailed information about the context in which that communication occurs. They are going to show us how our adolescents perceive the same reality that we share, what elements of that world that we have presented to them and left them as an inheritance, seem ironic, ridiculous, absurd, enough to dismantle them in a humorous way and build their own world.

There are countless of them and as is the case with any element generated on the internet, as we write these lines, countless new ones have already been generated. We leave you a selection of those who, due to their expressive capacity, have become the most iconic on the internet.

Baby Cha-Cha-Cha or Dancing Baby

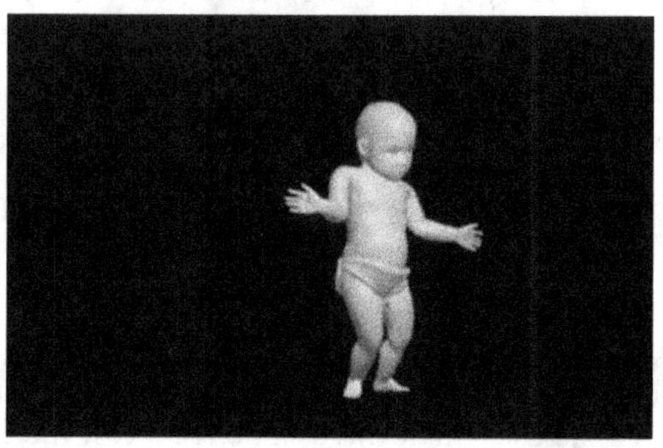

It was the first meme that went viral, back in 1996. At that time, the Internet was not widespread enough to go viral, but television was still very strong and this meme became popular thanks to the series Ally McBeal, in which It appeared as a hallucination suffered by the protagonist.

'Hide the pain Harold' or "the man with the most disturbing smile in the world"

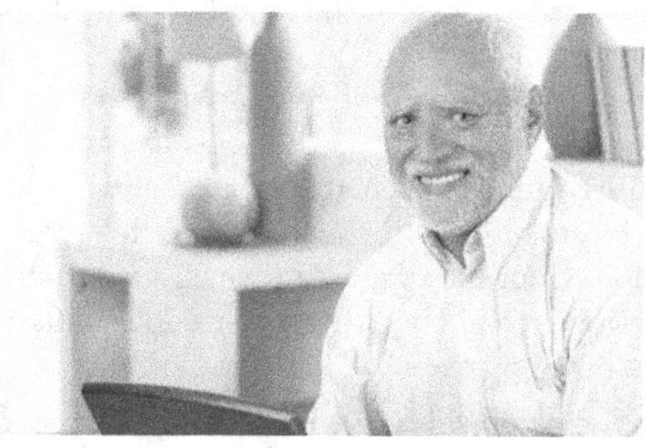

This famous man is, in reality, a retired Hungarian engineer, whose fake smile fits perfectly to describe any situation in which social circumstances force us to appear happy or happy.

Disaster Girl

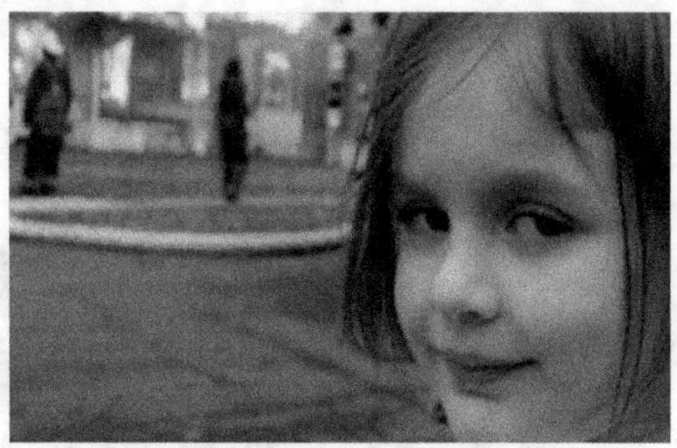

Zoë Roth became world famous when her maliciously smiling face in front of a burning building won a contest in 2007. Since then, it is the most used to describe any situation with hidden intentions. By the way, Zoë never revealed if she really had anything to do with the fire.

Fry from Futurama

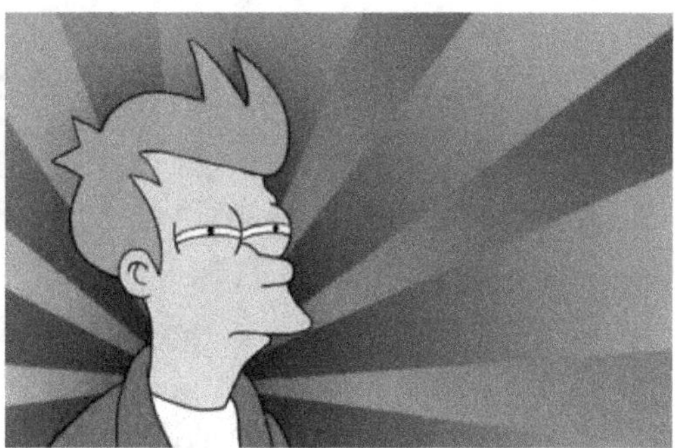

This meme of the Futurama series character with squinting eyes is used to express skepticism, suspicion, or confusion. But it is also used for the opposite, that is, to reflect a luminous moment of understanding. Something like that, like the Mona Lisa of memes, who depending on how you look at her, understands or doubts.

This is fine

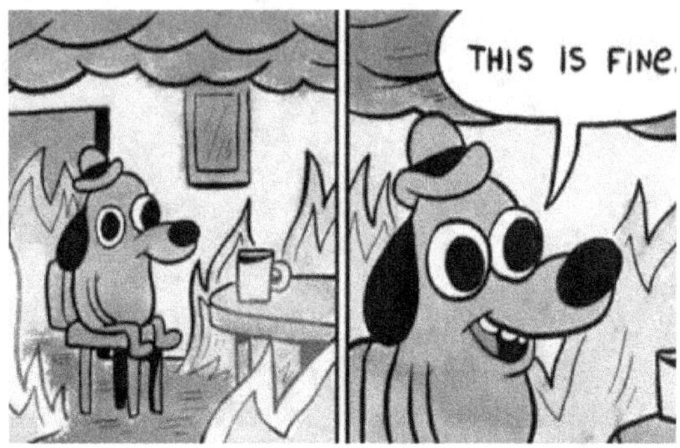

This dog in flames is used to represent situations where things are going wrong, but one is optimistic or tries to ignore the bad. It is also dedicated to those people who, because they are too positive, show little empathy and never see seriousness in what happens to us.

Distracted boyfriend

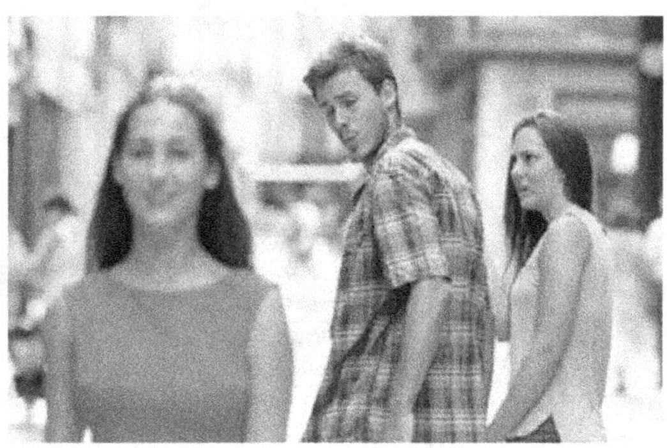

The image speaks for itself. But beyond its love context, this meme is used to represent situations in which someone shows interest in something new while ignoring something or someone with whom they have any type of relationship. They could be, for example, soccer players deciding on the team they are going to sign for instead of staying with their usual club, or politicians forgetting about their government partners and approaching positions with the opposition.

Pepe the frog

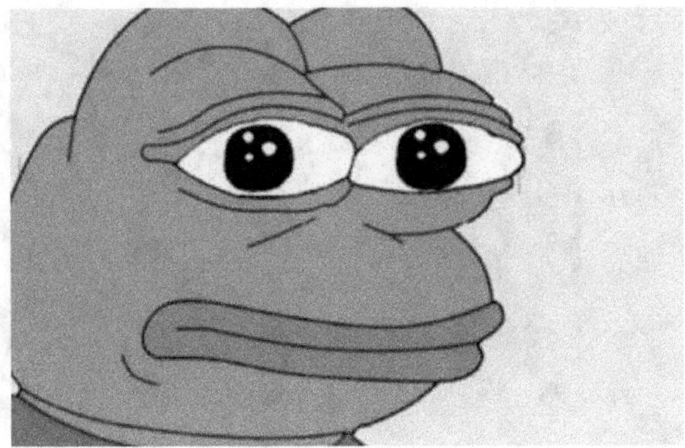

This character from a comic called Boy's Club became a widely used meme for his expressive ability. It is associated with different expressions and moods, which it reflects very accurately.

Doge

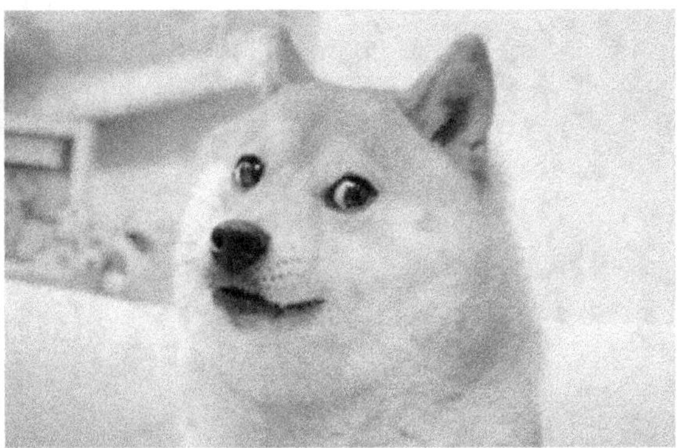

Poorly written text is often added to this image of a Shiba Inu in order to express emotions that can also be very diverse, such as surprise, happiness or confusion. His expressive ability is what has made him one of the most iconic memes on the internet.

Surprised Pikachu

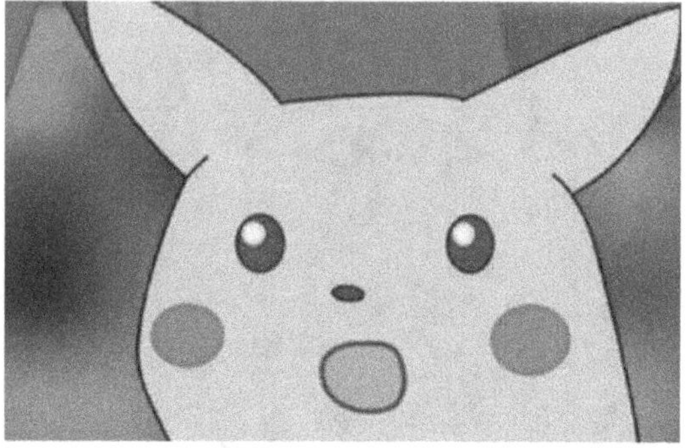

The famous Pokémon series character with a surprised expression is used when something obvious or predictable surprises. Humor lies, therefore, in the fact that the person who uses it perfectly stages his innocence or ignorance about the topic being talked about.

Woman yelling at a cat

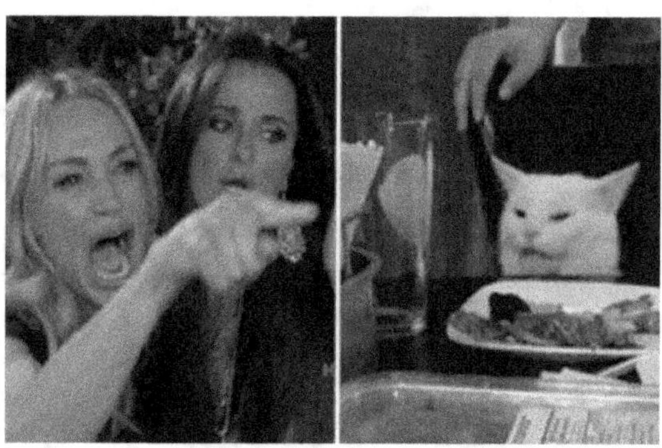

This funny meme is used to represent a situation in which someone is expressing a disproportionate opinion or complaint, losing their manners, while the other party reacts with bewilderment or indifference.

Philosoraptor

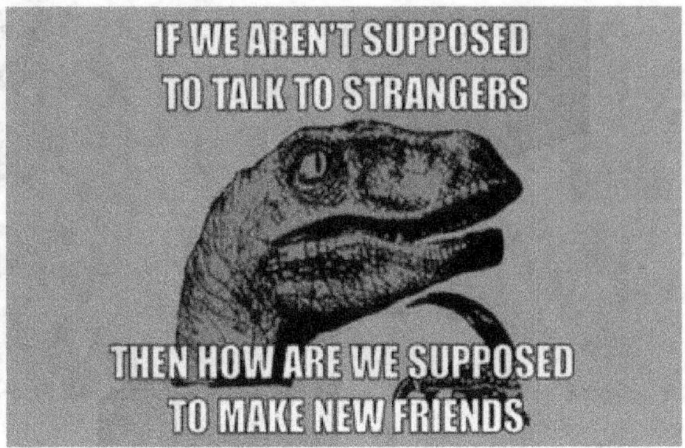

This image of a velociraptor with a thoughtful or reflective pose is usually combined with a question or an ironic philosophical statement, which plays with the concept that a prehistoric dinosaur is immersed in the contemplation of life or existential problems.

Success kid

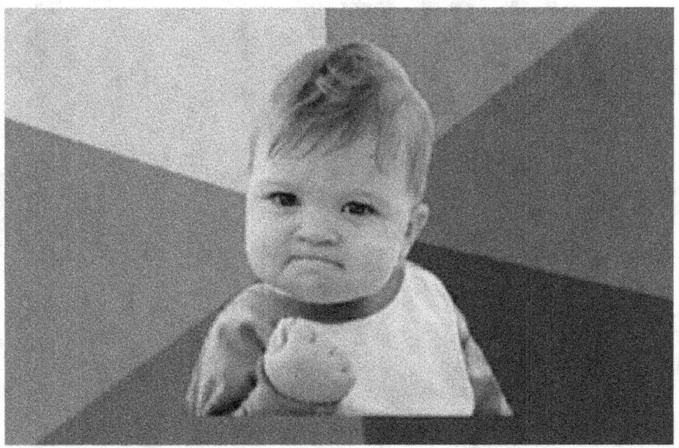

This gesture says it all. And coming from someone still so young, it is used to talk about those everyday achievements or triumphs, no matter how small they may be. For example, if we have started a diet and lose some weight. There are so many small everyday victories and the child's face is so expressive that this meme has become the favorite of many.

Evil Kermit

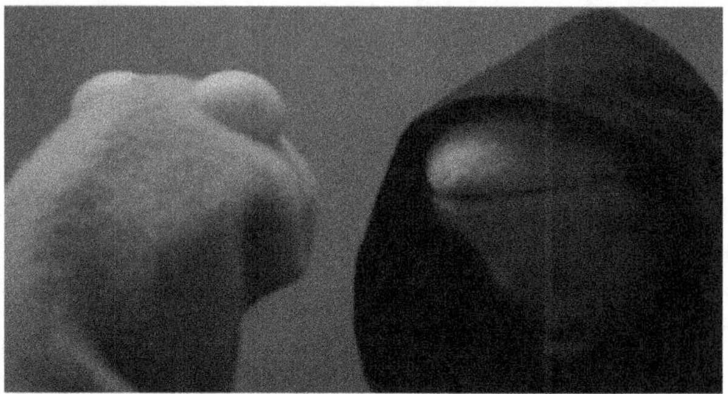

This meme humorously represents the internal struggle that we all sometimes feel, between making a responsible decision or succumbing to temptation or desire.

Roll safe

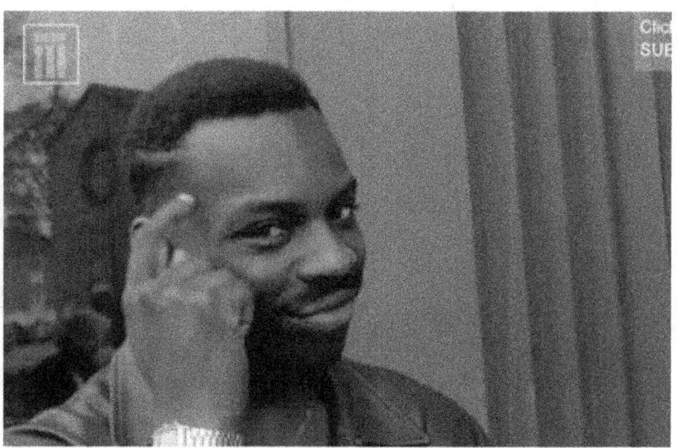

This meme is used when we propose a solution to a somewhat counterproductive problem. For example, someone may suggest that, to save water, we turn our underwear inside out instead of putting them in the wash.

We could continue with them, since we confess that it has been the most fun part of our investigation. But to exemplify their relevance in the description of the social context in which they occur, they are already sufficient.

We leave this chapter here, which together with the previous ones, closes the investigation into the sources of linguistic influence that have to do with Internet culture, the main one in terms of the generation and use of Slang. But slang also draws on another powerful source of linguistic influence: popular culture, especially musical culture, which has its own particularities. Let's go with the music somewhere else.

5. MUSIC SLANG

Classroom diary.

Tuesday, 9:00 in the morning. I go to class excited. Today it's time to talk about one of my favorite topics: Renaissance art. I have a well-designed session with which to convey my passion for Michelangelo, Botticelli or Da Vinci. But as I approach the hallway, something tells me that it's not going to be the day I expected: Taylor Swift and her Love Story have taken over my classroom.

Lola is a very vital student, although somewhat shy. It is beautiful to work with her, because when you help her overcome her shyness, her strength drives her to do great work. Teachers rarely have the privilege of participating in the fruits of the work we do with students. Normally, our job consists of sowing, but not harvesting, and I must confess that, at least personally, when I am lucky enough to meet one of these students, who remind you of the importance and beauty of our vocation made profession, I I get a special affection. Perhaps because of that bias and because I was surprised to see her so uninhibited and so happy, I did not react with the severity that the moment demanded when I found her standing on a table, with Taylor Swift's music coming out at full volume through the classroom speakers. , singing and dancing accompanied by Judith and Alejandra, who cheered with amusement.

"We have tickets, teacher!" "They let us go see her!" She got off the table and came running to give me a hug to make me share in her joy, unaware of the inappropriateness of the situation she was causing with her happiness overflowing from her. Within that lack of control, everything flowed with surprising normality, as if this explosion of joy seemed justified and natural to everyone.

"Tickets for what, Lola?" I managed to say.

"Who will it be for, teacher! To see Taylor Swift, who is coming to Spain!"

"I'm very happy for you, Lola, congratulations! But come on, dismantle this scenario for me, we have to talk about artists, yes, but about other more important ones," I said, trying to recompose the situation, letting that beginning of tomorrow pass as normal. that no one seemed to care, except loveYo.

"More important? There's no one more important than Taylor Swift!" Lola said.

"Yes, there is. Rosalía!" Alejandra immediately responded.

"What are you saying! They're BTS," Sara added, joining the conversation.

"The BTS? But K-Pop is only music for girls. Give me a little bit of Maluma and Bad Bunny and I'll take away everything else," said Rubén, with his usual tone from which he has nothing to learn. because he doubts nothing, despite being only fifteen years old.

"Shut up! You wish you were as good as them," Sara replied, normally temperate, but making it clear that this topic was very important to her, almost sacred.

"If there is no respect, there is no debate! Everyone in their place or out of class!" I had no choice but to intervene bravely to calm things down.

"Sorry, teacher, it's not because we're lacking, but some artists who have been dead for centuries... it's really lazy. What do we care about them? Understand that we like to talk more about our own," Judith wanted to mediate, acting as she was, from a magnificent classroom representative.

Without meaning to, Judith had just thrown me the life preserver that allowed me to return to the ship. She had to take the opportunity to regain the helm and prevent the class from sinking. "Why are you so sure that you like yours better? Look, I don't understand much about music, much less current music, but I do know something more about art in general. For example, I know that what you I like it, it has a lot to do with what I was going to explain to you, because when art is good, it touches the same fibers that move us as human beings, regardless of whether we are human beings of the 21st century or the 11th century. You have all highlighted me current music artists and yet many of you mention very different styles. What makes you more hooked on a specific style, a specific artist over another?" She had just returned the question to them. Now I set the tempos.

"Well in my case, because they express exactly what I feel," Valeria rightly commented, after a few seconds of pause.

"Fair," "it's like that," "lit," "yes to everything," "it represents me," the audience cheered.

"What if I told you that the same thing you feel, whatever it is, was felt by others before you? What if the artists who once felt it, left us an eternal work, capable of empathizing with us even today? today? Sometimes you only need a few notions to understand it, as happens with your musical styles, and thus ensure that its messages become understandable. Ensure that its messages reach us with all their force. And when you manage to reach you one of the great artists of any time, and their work makes your hair stand on end, you will understand why I tell you that they are more important than those that you simply like.

I was comfortable. I thought I had settled the debate with my final rant... but no. Nico launched a derivative that moved away from the emotional, and provided a much less elaborate argument, but with which he managed to get the class on his side.

"Bah teacher, it's not the same. Feeling love and things like that may be. But who do you fall in love with... Let's see, I'm sure they also liked the hot chicks... the pretty girls. But the ones that are "You see them in museums, I don't like them. They have nothing to do with the ones that appear in the music videos or the ones I think of when I listen to my songs," he said.

"Fair", "it's like that", "lit", "yes to everything", "it represents me", the audience cheered again.

"They have nothing to do with each other? They have everything to do with each other! Or do you think that what seems beautiful to you now is not conditioned by what we have defined as beautiful over the centuries? Let's do an experiment. Veronica , you who draw so well.

Go out to the board and draw the man and the woman who describe those songs, those people who keep us awake, who make us fall in love and break our hearts. Draw them according to the descriptions that the companions".

While Verónica fought with the chalk trying to faithfully reflect what a chicken coop of voices was telling her (with some happy discrepancies), I was preparing two images: that of David, by Miguel Ángel Buonarroti, and that of The Birth of Venus, by Sandro Botticelli. With them and with Verónica's drawings, we built a comparative class in which we questioned whether what seemed beautiful to them was genuine or whether they were influenced, even in the 21st century, by the masculine and feminine ideals of beauty defined in the Renaissance canons. of the 15th and 16th centuries, which in turn recovered those defined in the Classical world, in Greco-Latin culture, as shown in The Vitruvian Man by Leonardo Da Vinci, based on the study of the proportions of the architect Vitruvius, from Ancient Rome. .

"It's been a really aesthetic class, teacher. One day we have to do it the other way around, because I'm sure you're also influenced by the artists we like." Nico left me thinking about his words all afternoon. To his " aesthetic class" that hammered in my head, and to the meaning of his statement. Could it be true that I was influenced by artists that were not mine, those that I do not usually follow and even those that I would be able to affirm that they do not suit me? Almost unconsciously, I checked my Spotify music selection. Although my Rock classics and some touches of Jazz predominated, I had been adding other new songs from current groups that I was completely unaware of, but whose compositions, recommended by the application's algorithm, I had liked until I saved them in my selection of favorite songs. It was time to recognize that Nico had indeed hit the nail on the head.

The subsequent conversations with Borja Núñez to prepare the book clarified a lot about this to me. It is not only we who choose which aspects of culture we want to enjoy, but the cultural context in which we move contributes a lot to our way of being, because in our relationships with others, we are also influenced by them and we try to find shared elements that promote our links. And that is especially noticeable in the way we communicate. That is, it is especially noticeable in the Slang.

By focusing on it, we have reducedinThis chapter, exclusively to music, the cultural elements that influence adolescents. Of course, there are many other elements that could be talked about, but they are much less relevant in the construction of slang. Neither fashion, nor cinema, nor series generate terms that resonate among young people, beyond some limited term catchphrase, only valid during the duration of the film, series or fashion that is being followed. They are still young enough for literature, painting, sculpture or architecture to move them like a song can. They need to continue training to have the keys that allow them to understand them, as well as experiences associated with adult life to seek answers and consolation in them. And if there are other creative elements that influence them, generated by some of their favorite artists who are now called "content creators", they manifest themselves through video games, video channels and social networks, which we have already analyzed. It is For this reason, it seems appropriate to limit the cultural influence that adolescent slang suffers to that produced by the different musical styles they listen to.

Indeed, there are many slang terms for teenagers who are born in music. And due to its universality, they tend to be terms born in English speaking, since the most international artists sing in this language and, like them, the terms are recognized and used by teenagers from all over the world, who follow them. Some of them, as an example, may be the following:

Bae:
It comes from the English phrase 'Before anyone else'. It is therefore an affectionate word to refer to a partner or loved one. "My 'bae' took me to dinner last night"
Dope:
It means great or impressive. You may hear someone say "that song is really 'dope'".
Flex:
It means to show or boast about something, often related to achievements, possessions, or abilities. For example, she is 'flexing' her new sneakers.
FOMO:
Acronym for Fear of Missing Out. This term is used to describe the fear of missing out on an exciting experience that

others are having. "I don't want to stay home, I have 'FOMO'."

GOAT:

Acronym for Greatest of All Time. It is used to describe someone or something that is considered the best of all time. For example, "Taylor Swift is the 'GOAT' of music."

Lit:

Although in Spain it is used as an abbreviation for "literal", in reality this adjective from English is used to describe something that is exciting or great. For example, "last night's party was very lit."

Lit as:

Similar to "lit", but used to express that something is extremely exciting or good. "That party was 'lit as hell'."

Squad:

It refers to a group of close friends. It is common to hear teenagers say things like "I went out with my 'squad' to the movies."

Turn up:

Used to express fun or excitement. You may hear someone say "let's 'turn up' tonight at the party."

Vibes:

It refers to the atmosphere or general atmosphere of a place or time. For example, "the vibes at the concert were incredible."

We could make a much longer list, since there are many terms used in adolescent slang that are born in music. But if the fact of knowing this Slang has to bring us closer to knowing our teenage sons and daughters better, what we must focus on is knowing the Slang of the different musical styles that they have chosen as their music, since the particularities of each one will help us. They will in turn help us to know the particularities of our daughter or our son. The most popular styles among teenagers today are Pop (and its Korean version, K-Pop), Reggaeton and other Latin rhythms, and Hip-Hop. There are many other styles that are still valid, such as Rock or Electronic Music, and others that have a lot of local strength, such as Country in rural environments in the USA or Flamenco, here in Spain. However, to limit the infinite number of terms born from all types of music, we will focus our study on the Slang derived from the most listened to musical styles.

The most popular of all among teenagers is Pop music, due, above all, to its catchy melodies and accessible lyrics. Artists like our protagonist Taylor Swift, Justin Bieber and Ariana Grande are highly appreciated in this genre, but in this case, precisely because of that universality, the Pop genre does not have a specific Slang as distinctive as other musical styles. There are numerous words and phrases that have become popular in adolescent slang that have their roots in Pop, but none of them tend to be used in small groups, that link their followers and can give us information about what they feel and how they want to be. . They are very popular terms, so much so that they go beyond the musical context to become something much broader, in the so-called Pop culture, which permeates many other areas of our lives. We take as an example the following:

Fan:
This term is widely used to describe someone who is a passionate fan of a popular artist, group, or television series.
Fandom:
It is a community of fans who share a common interest in an artist, group or franchise. For example, the "fandom" of a Pop band.
Hit:
It is used to describe a song or movie that becomes very popular and successful.
Influencer:
It is a person who has a large presence on social networks and who can influence the opinions and choices of other teenagers. This applies to Pop music figures and other content creators.
Playlist:
It is a list of selected songs that are created for a specific occasion, to share with friends or simply for personal enjoyment.
Selfie:
It's a word that has become ubiquitous in teen culture thanks to the practice of taking photos of oneself.
Shippear (Ship):
It refers to the action of supporting or desiring a romantic relationship between two fictional characters or two

celebrities, often from Pop music. It comes from the term "relationship" in English.

Stream:

It refers to the action of playing music or online content, which is common among teenagers to listen to their favorite songs.

Throwback (TBT):

It is a term used to refer to something from the past, such as a retro song or fashion. Teens often post photos and memories as part of "Throwback Thursday" (TBT) on social media.

Viral:

It is used to describe something that spreads quickly online, such as a song, video, or trend.

It is very common during adolescence for our daughter or son to show interest in this type of music. At least, it will be the first one I access as "her music" from her. She is happy, positive and very danceable, which makes her the most chosen among teenagers to enjoy free time with friends, at parties or going clubbing. But apart from personal enjoyment, being a fan of Pop music has some other advantages. For example, its lyrics full of romantic feelings allow teenagers to accompany their first experiences with love and more easily express their emotions in their first crushes and breakups. But if there is an advantage that we would like to highlight about Pop music, it is mainly that by being so popular among teenagers of all ages (also among those over thirty, forty and fifty), this type of music becomes a point of intergenerational connection that allows us, if we free ourselves from complexes, to share the same passion with fathers and mothers with daughters and sons.

Of course, the fact that it is the most listened to musical genre also entails some disadvantages. For example, it is difficult in adolescence to find the path that defines us, even more so if that path takes us away from the group of friends that we would like to continue accompanying us. That's why in music, it's common to follow popular trends instead of choosing the one we really like. And to this we must add that, to fully fit in with the group, they may feel the need to invest not inconsiderable sums of money in dressing and acting according to the canons of their favorite artists, especially if the group also does so.

friendships in which they move. Trying to talk to them about it is usually a source of friction, since it is very difficult for us to understand the needs of the other: those of belonging to the group that the adolescent has and those of correctly investing what is available in the domestic economy that we adults have. There is no recipe that works with this, if there were, adolescence would not be the wonderful challenge that it is. The messages we try to convey to them will resonate, and they will even replicate them with their own children, but only when the adolescent virus has been completely cured. Everything involves having patience in moments of conflict and knowing how to generate, enjoy and value moments of connection with them, which through music can be easier for us than with new technologies.

Without moving away from Pop music, in recent years, music of this style has been strongly joined by Korean Pop music, known as K-Pop, which has gained presence especially among the adolescent public. Groups like BTS, BLACKPINK or TWICE are iconic in this genre. Of course, unlike Pop, K-Pop has its own Slang, with terms that are used by followers and artists of this type of music, creating a community among them. The most representative are the following:

Aegyo:
It is a term used to describe a loving and close attitude or behavior. Some K-Pop idols display "aegyo" in their interactions with fans.

Bias:
This term refers to the favorite member of a K-Pop group. Fans often have a "bias" within a group, meaning they have a favorite member.

Comeback:
In K-Pop, a "comeback" does not refer to a return in the literal sense, but to the release of new music or a new album by a group or artist. Comebacks are often exciting times for fans.

Debut:
It is the moment when a new group or artist is officially presented in the music industry. It is an important moment in the career of a group and its fans.

Fan Service:
It refers to the gestures or actions that artists perform to please their fans. This may include close interactions, gifts, greetings,

and other loving gestures toward fans.

Fanchant:

It is a choreographed chant that fans perform during live performances to show their support for the group or artist. "Fanchants" often include members' names and other specific verses.

Lightstick:

They are light-up devices that fans bring to K-Pop concerts. Each group usually has their own official "light stick" with a specific design that fans wave during live performances.

Maknae:

He is the youngest member of a group. This term is used to identify the youngest member and is often shown affection and protection by the other members.

Stan:

It is derived from the Eminem song "Stan" and has become a word used to describe passionate and dedicated fans of a group or artist. To "fan" someone means to be a loyal fan.

Visual:

It is the member who is considered the most attractive or aesthetically pleasing in a group. This term is often used to describe the member who is seen as the most handsome.

If our daughter or son shows interest in this type of music, we can discover many facets of them that might otherwise go unnoticed, or understand some others that we did not understand when they occurred in other contexts. For example, a teenager who likes K-Pop tends to be an open-minded person, capable of exploring and appreciating cultures different from their own. Likewise, he reflects a creative personality, both in form and substance, since the songs of this musical genre combine music, images and a narrative with very elaborate stories. They are also very sensitive people, for whom K-Pop music helps them connect and allows them to open up, both on an individual level, empathizing with the stories told in the songs, and on a social level, connecting with a community. of fans with whom to share this passion.

However, as always when a passion becomes excessive, if the only thing our teenage daughter or son shows interest in is everything related to the K-Pop universe, they could be using it as an emotional refuge, which, far from allowing them to open up, make him take refuge. Her followers tend to be, as we say, especially empathetic and sensitive, which is fantastic for connecting with others, but only if we manage not to feel overwhelmed. If the social environment surpasses us, we tend to isolate ourselves. To counteract this, K-Pop music itself, through the lyrics of its songs, can help us find those positive examples that serve as a mirror in which to look at ourselves to overcome those situations in which we feel more insecure. Getting closer to this music, listening to its songs, speaking its slang and even going to a concert together, can help us connect with our children and better influence their growth.

Along with Pop music in all its versions, music labeled as Latin is sweeping among teenagers, especially Reggaeton, which in recent years has gained popularity around the world and attracts teenagers regardless of their place of origin. Artists like Bad Bunny, J Balvin and Rosalía are leading figures in this genre, which of course, also has its own slang. Some of the most used terms globally are the following:

Street map:
It is a term used to describe life on the street, the experiences that occur there and that are reflected in their songs.
Demobow:
It is the characteristic rhythm of Reggaeton. It is a repeating drum pattern and is an essential part of reggaeton music.
Hard/Hard:
In Reggaeton, "dura" or "duro" is used to describe someone who is brave, strong or talented. It can refer to a person or a song that is perceived as powerful.
Flow:
It refers to the style and way an artist presents themselves in a song. Each reggaeton player can have their own distinctive "flow."
Street flow:
It refers to a style of Reggaeton that focuses on themes related to life on the street, fighting and overcoming obstacles.
Latin Flow:
It is used to describe the style and influence of Latin culture on Reggaeton music, characterized by vibrant rhythms and

dances.

Perreo:

It refers to a sensual dance style that is often associated with Reggaeton. The dance involves provocative movements, almost always performed by women, and is very common at parties and video clips of this musical style.

Caught/turned on:

In the context of Reggaeton, "prendo" or "prendida" refers to being excited or enthusiastic. It can be used to describe a lively party or an excited person. It derives from the translation of the much more widespread term "lit."

Trap:

Subgenre of reggaeton that often features darker and more thematic lyrics that they call "street" lyrics. It combines elements of Reggaeton with Hip-Hop influences.

Tusa:

It is a word that means sadness or disappointment in Reggaeton slang. The song "Tusa" by Karol G and Nicki Minaj popularized this term.

If our children are moved by these Latin rhythms, we have before us an energetic teenager who enjoys dancing and can channel through it, an impetus that could otherwise be difficult to contain. But if our cultural roots also have an origin that fits with the label of Latin, Reggaeton and other rhythms so called serve to link today's young people with their tradition, with their previous generations, creating a strong feeling of community, which is gathers around partying and dancing to share moments of joy with their loved ones.

Of course, especially Reggaeton is a musical genre whose lyrics include recurring themes of violence, drugs, sex and, above all, a great hypersexualization of women. Many of their songs promote gender stereotypes and sexist attitudes, which can condition the perception and behavior of our teenage daughters and sons in their first relationships. Do we therefore censor this type of music? We believe that there is no need to be alarmist if our children are well informed and understand the risks of the lyrics of the music that moves them. Many of my students enjoy these songs without their attitude towards others having been negatively transformed. Even using myself as an example, since I have always liked Rock and it is surely something that many of us share, I have listened to countless songs in which all types of drugs were advocated, without having become addicted or simply in consumer. I have never tried them nor would I do so again.

Beyond the jokes, if we spend time talking to our children about these risks, we ensure that their self-esteem does not involve relying on them and knowing that they are well informed of the possible consequences, the "bad messages" that music of any genre can transmit, are simply limited to the musical context in which they occur, without having to be reproduced in the rest of the facets of our daughters and sons' lives.

And like the previous styles, Hip-Hop is the last of the musical genres that we want to highlight as one of the most influential in slang. Artists like Drake, Kendrick Lamar and Billie Eilish are having a huge impact on young people. And from his lyrics, many of the terms that have enriched adolescent slang emerge, such as:

Beef:
It originally referred to the rivalry or dispute between rappers, often expressed in song lyrics. Now it is used in a broader sense, to refer to any type of discussion or enmity.
Bling-Bling:
It refers to jewelry and expensive and flashy accessories and accessories, often worn by rappers and Hip-Hop artists.
Dope:
It is used to describe something that is great, incredible or impressive.
Flex/Flexin':
It is used to describe the display of success, wealth or confidence. "Flexin'" is the act of showing off or showing off.
Freestylin':
It is the action of improvising lyrics or rhymes on the spot, often in an impromptu rap competition.
Fresh:
It is used to praise something that is new, modern and elegant. In Hip-Hop, "fresh" is often associated with style and fashion.
Hater:
It is someone who criticizes or envies others, often unfairly. The term is used in Hip-Hop to describe people who express

hatred or envy towards artists.

Homie:
It is an informal term used to refer to a close friend or colleague. It is very common in Hip-Hop slang.

Lyrical Genius:
It refers to a rapper or artist with an exceptional talent for creating intelligent and creative lyrics.

Mic Drop:
It refers to a dramatic gesture in which someone drops a microphone after giving an outstanding performance, often used as a powerful final statement, in which there is no right of reply.

Squad:
It is a close group of friends or colleagues. It is commonly used to describe your social group.

Swag:
It refers to someone's personal style, confidence, and attitude. In Hip-Hop culture, having "swag" is a desired quality.

Turnt:
It is a term used to describe someone who is excited and ready to have fun at a party or event.

A teenager who likes Hip-Hop, he is saying about himself that he is a sensitive and creative person, who finds in music and rhymes the way to express his emotions and thoughts. He is also a committed person, who shows interest in what is happening around him, developing a social conscience that serves as inspiration for lyrics that are often protesting and denouncing. And the fact of being so critical of their environment makes them be demanding of themselves, highly valuing authenticity.. Tratnto show themselves as they are on that path of personal growth, which in adolescence tends to become complicated when what the reference group is looking for clouds what one is looking for oneself. But in the case of Hip-Hop, the search for what is genuine is something shared. It does not generate isolation but quite the opposite: a community that shares not only music, but much broader cultural manifestations, which are usually grouped under the name of urban art.

However, the recipes that appear in the lyrics of their songs to resolve all the negative things they denounce are not always positive.

In them, sexual, violence or drug themes are frequently used, which can promote negative stereotypes, such as the justification of violence to solve problems, or drug consumption and sex as rewards and goals to achieve.

But as was the case with Reggaeton or any other musical genre that is inspired by intimate experiences or those lived on the street, apart from day-to-day routines (which are much less inspiring), we must remember that it is only about of music. If there was a real danger, our children would show signs of some other elements. One of them, which it is advisable to be very aware of, as it is a clear indicator of knowing the danger well and not showing interest due to the need to appear in front of their groups of friends, is the concrete and specific Slang that is created and used to hide them. Issues related to drugs, gambling and sports betting, risks to adolescent sexual intimacy or eating disorders (ED), have a specific Slang to communicate without being detected. It's dangerous Slang.

6. DANGEROUS SLANG

Surely this is a chapter for reference only, without the information contained herein being needed on a day-to-day basis. We are convinced that the love and concern you feel for your children, which has made them interested in this book, is the best barrier to prevent your teenage son or daughter from finding themselves immersed in a dangerous situation.

But, even if it is not, the risks around it exist. And as our children grow and their world apart from their parents grows with them, the probability that they will encounter these risks becomes greater. If we have transmitted love to them, we have created a relationship in which they can feel confident, we have educated them to understand what is right and what is not, and they have received the necessary information about the risks they will encounter and their consequences. , we can trust that they have the necessary tools to overcome or overcome them. Our teenagers are excellent people who will surely know how to get along without us, thanks to us. But if the restlessness does not leave us completely, it is because, although excellent, they are still adolescents, that is, people with a desire to discover new things, to experiment with what their environment offers them and with their own body. People, furthermore, who need to self-affirm the acceptance of their group. And both group pressure and the desire to experiment are powerful arguments that can make our son or daughter act incorrectly and fool around with some of the risks. If we add to this cocktail that, when they first come into contact with these risks, they feel ashamed or believe that we are not going to understand them and therefore, we are not going to know or want to help them, they will probably want to hide them from us, making the situation worse. One of the most common ways to hide them from us is to use codes that they know we cannot understand, to talk about them without giving themselves away. If necessary, we believe that knowing this Slang can help us know when to talk to our children without letting them slip through lies, or to go to the professional that we consider can best help us in this situation.

Dangerous slang is not adolescent slang per se, but social slang, that is, it is used by people of any age to refer to these risks, hiding them from the rest of society. They are not common in adolescent slang, in fact, I have not resisted asking several of them to my children, who were completely unaware of them (fortunately). But without being habitual, adolescents are permeable to them and even if it is only for a minority, even if it is only one, our daughter or our son, it seems appropriate to offer them in this book, the codes that are used to be able to attend as soon as possible. possible any attempt at risk that could condition them.

What risks are we talking about? In adolescence there are many of those that experts warn us about. Several of them, such as addiction to video games, mobile phones or harassment, especially through social networks (cyberbullying), we have already mentioned in previous chapters. We will not dwell on them further, since they are not associated with a specific Slang. In this chapter we want to focus on others that are less frequent, but unfortunately exist among adolescents: practices that involve a loss of intimacy and even sexual blackmail, initiation into drugs and addiction to sports betting and games of chance. All of them accompanied by their own codes. Along with them, we also want to focus on eating disorders (ED), which, although they do not have extensive Slang, hide behind all kinds of horrible information that advises young people on how to continue losing weight. And unfortunately, this risk is much more common among adolescents.

Loss of intimacy and sexual blackmail.

Through social networks, there are sexual initiation practices that cause these types of situations. They are even used by pedophiles, who, with a false profile, pose as teenagers to obtain material with explicit content. It's grooming.

But without contact with a pedophile, sexting is practiced among adolescents themselves, consisting of sending intimate photos or videos to other people. Sometimes, this risky practice is aggravated by the blackmail to which the person about whom we have material of sexual content is subjected, which is known as sextortion. These online encounters could end up in in-person encounters, which would add many more risks to these situations.

To request this type of material, suggest meetings and warn of the presence or surveillance of parents, specific Slang is used based on the following terms:

121:
It means chatting privately.
53Xor CU46:
We meet to have sex
9, CD9, Code 9:
The parents are nearby.
99:
The parents are far away.
A3:
Anytime, anywhere, anywhere.
F2F:
Offer to video chat or meet in person (face to face).
GNOC:
It means "get naked in front of the camera."
GYPO:
It means "take off your pants."
KPC:
Keep parents off guard.
LMIRL:
Let's meet in real life
MOS/POS:
mom/dad are watching (looking over your shoulder)
Netflix and chill:
Originally, this referred to watching a movie and spending time together, but now this phrase can also be a proposition

to have sex.
Smash:
Have casual sex
Stalker:
Person who excessively reviews another's information on networks, as a form of harassment or persecution.
Sugarpic:
It is the request for a suggestive photo.
TDTM:
Talk dirty to Me.
WTTP:
Do you want to exchange photos?

Initiation into drugs

Without going into assessing the type of harmful or illegal substance that adolescents access, nor attempting to prioritize the seriousness of their consumption, something that we believe corresponds to you, the terms used to refer to any of them and the context in which which are usually common, are the following:

1174:
See you at the party (with wild party connotations).
420:
Relating to marijuana and its consumption.
Blue boogers:
Snort Adderall or Ritalin.
CID:
Acids, but also drugs in general.
Dayger:
Party during the day
Dospa:
Sharing a joint between two people, although it can also refer to hooking up with two different people in the same night.
Plug:
It is used to talk about someone who can obtain alcohol, drugs or illegal substances in general.
Function/Func:
Party

High:
Indicates being drugged or under the influence of a substance.
Jai:
Get really drunk.
Lit:
We have already seen it referring to something exciting or entertaining, but it can also be used to talk about being under the influence of drugs.
Molly, X:
The two ways of referring to ecstasy.
Party favors:
It can refer to drugs or substances consumed at parties.
Pharming:
The act of going into medicine cabinets to find drugs to get high.
Rager:
Big party
Just relax:
small party
Robo-tripping:
Consume cough syrup to get high.
Sloshed:
to be drunk
Speed, crank, uppers, Crystal, Tina:
The different ways of referring to methamphetamine
Throw Down:
to have a party
Turnt:
Being high or drunk (formerly "turnt up")
Go lacasito, go doraemon, go tinkiwinki:
Basically, he/she is drunk.
Vaping:
Referring to the use of electronic devices to consume substances, often nicotine or THC.
Wasted:
It refers to being very drunk or high.
White lady:
This is what cocaine and heroin are called.

Addiction to sports betting and gambling

Gambling, slot machines and betting on events of any kind, mainly sports, have always been prohibited by law for minors. Its design, designed to attract and engage with stimuli of all kinds, together with the negative consequences that this addiction has for the economic and social situation of the person who falls into its networks, have made us agree as a society on the fact that limit them exclusively to adult users. The fact oftolerateAmong adults, it already generates less consensus, with gambling being legal in many places, but a practice that is persecuted and punished in many others. Going to a gaming room, placing bets or spending all day at the slot machine in a bar were socially reprehensible behaviors, which limited addiction to those people who managed to hide it and those who no longer cared that no one saw them. because no one had them anymore.

But the facilities offered by the Internet and mobile devices to put at our fingertips what we want at all times, and also to be able to do so with the necessary privacy so as not to generate disapproval, have multiplied the cases of gambling addiction today. And this has also happened with our minors. A violation of the very few security measures of gaming applications (sometimes it is enough to simply indicate the date of birth and affirm that you are an adult), has caused many of our young people and adolescents to have developed serious problems with gambling addiction. .

Being minors, their family social network is usually resistant enough that, with appropriate professional attention, the situation can be reversed. But as with any evil that can threaten us, the sooner it is detected, the more likely it is to solve it. Therefore, we consider it important that you know some of the most used terms when using games of chance and sports betting, in order to prevent as much as possible:

All in:
It refers to betting everything you have on a single bet, usually in the context of gambling.
Banker:
Selection of a bet in which you have a lot of confidence and is combined with another riskier bet to increase the profit.

Bankroll:
The amount of money a person has available to bet or play.
Betting the farm:
Betting a large amount of money, similar to betting the farm.
Bookie:
Betting house.
Cash:
Available balance in a betting house.
Chalk:
Bet with a high probability of being successful.
Chasing:
It means continuing to bet or gamble in an attempt to recover what has been lost.
Dog:
Bet on the underdog.
Dutching:
Divide an amount of money between several options of the same event to diversify the risk.
Evens:
Bet even or odds 2.00, with which you get double what you bet.
Get rich quick scheme:
A plan or idea that promises quick and significant profits.
Green:
Term used to refer to bills, usually dollars.
High roller / Whale:
A person who bets large amounts of money.
Jackpot:
The largest possible prize in a game of chance.
Nap:
Maximum confidence bet made public by a professional forecaster.
Parlay:
Combined bet in which all predictions must be correct to win.
Penny Ante:
Betting small amounts of money, often on casual games.
Playing the odds:
Betting based on the odds of winning.
Pick:
Forecast.

Risky business:
It can refer to dangerous or risky activities.
ROI:
Return on investment. It is the indicator that measures the success of a tipster.
Stacks:
It can refer to piles of money or chips in a gambling game.
Tipster:
Sports predictor that recommends bets to other users.

Eating Disorders: Eating Disorders

The TCA Slang is only made up of two terms: #Ana and #Mia. Under the innocent appearance of these two tags with a woman's name, there are almost four million publications on social networks, according to the latest report from the Internet Quality Agency. #Ana and #Mia the code names to refer to anorexia and bulimia, used to opaquely share on social networks, horrible experiences, tricks and advice related to low-calorie eating, excuses for not eating and to hide it, and drastic ways to reduce the weight.

Unfortunately, this risk is quite common among our teenagers. In Spain, the Association against Anorexia and Bulimia (ACAB) carried out a study in 2019 among more than 750 students between 12 and 16 years old (from 1st to 4th ESO) from 14 educational centers. The result: 23% of these adolescents were at risk of suffering from anorexia or bulimia. And the trend today is upward.

We sincerely hope that you do not have to experience an eating disorder in your homes. If we suspect that something is happening, experts highlight the enormous importance of having a family lunch or dinner a day. An action as simple as this reduces the possibility of suffering from an eating disorder by up to 35%. When sitting at the table, having a mobile phone or tablet at hand should be avoided at all costs, so that they cannot interfere with the family conversation and the attachment and bond with the minor is strengthened. And as we always recommend, maintaining fluid communication with your children as much as possible and requesting professional help when you consider it necessary, are the best recipe we can follow to help our daughter or son overcome their eating disorder.

Much encouragement and strength if you find yourself struggling with any of the risks we have talked about. There are many success stories that should give us hope.

CONCLUSIONS: THE EXPERTS SPEAK

Conclusions of the protagonists

After several interviews with boys and girls between 10 and 17 years old, a first conclusionthat they transmit to usunanimously, it is clear: no, adults should not speak like teenagers do today. However, from these conversations, some exceptions to the use of their Slang can also be extracted, which it may be highly advisable to know for what they represent in themselves.

To fully understand what they want to tell us, it is best to read the transcripts of the interviews or listen to them directly thanks to the accompanying QR code. Since we did not request permission for its reproduction from the parents of the adolescents interviewed, we are going to transfer here the opinions of those who we know will not cause us legal problems: two of my children, Iván, 10 years old, and Dani, 12, and two nieces of Borja Núñez, Aitana, 14, and Ainhoa, 16 years old. They seem to us to be a very significant age sample and their opinions reflect the opinions expressed generally by the majority of the adolescents interviewed.

Youtube link:
https://acortar.link/wcdfzs

We start with my son Iván, who is still 10 years old, but is making leaps and bounds towards adolescence. He expressed himself this way:

Interviewer:"Hello Ivan. You're not a teenager yet, but you seem very clear about your position on the questions we're asking. Do you think that adults can talk like kids today?"
Ivan:"No".
Interviewer:"Why not?".
Ivan:"Well, there are two things why you can't be like today's children: because you don't get hit and because you're not used to it."
Interviewer:"What do you mean we're not used to it?"
Ivan:"Well, most of the time normal words would escape you."
Interviewer:"That is to say, we would mix your words with our words and the phrase would look strange. Is that?".
Ivan:"Yes, fair. It doesn't look natural. And besides, it doesn't hit you."
Interviewer:"But what do you mean he doesn't hit us?"
Ivan:"Well, your way of speaking doesn't match that of today."
Interviewer:"Do you mean that parents have to speak like parents for our own good, because we look bad if we try to speak differently?"
Ivan:"If that is. Your moment has already passed."
Interviewer:"Thank you very much for your opinions, Mr. Expert."
Ivan:"Okay."

It's curious. To avoid jealousy between siblings, we also interviewed my son Álvaro, 6 years old. It turns out that at that age they still don't see the problem with an adult speaking however they want. However, Iván, at 10, already defends that this should not be, and that statement becomes increasingly clearer as the interviewee gets older: Dani is more emphatic, and Aitana is even more so. This is how each of them expressed themselves:

Interviewer:"Well, Dani. I, who am your father, already know your answer, but still, we want to ask you to explain to us why you think we should not speak the way you speak."
Dani (12 years old):"You had a different Slang when you were young like we do now, and your turn has already passed. "Now it's our turn."
Interviewer:"How do you feel when you see an adult trying to

speak your slang?"

Dani:"Shame of others."

Interviewer:"Man, you used my language, how would you say it in yours?"

Dani:"Lache. "You are lazy."

Interviewer:"Is there any context in which you think we can express ourselves…"

Dani:"No!" (Interrupts me).

Interviewer:"None?".

Dani:"No!".

Interviewer:"For example, we are talking more seriously. You want to tell me something intimate and you're having a hard time finding the words… Could I use yours to make the communication flow better?"

Dani: "No! Worse. Much worse".

Interviewer:"Okay. You have made your position clear. Thank you".

Dani:"Bye bye".

Dani appears dry and blunt, but that is not only due to his age, but also to the trust that exists between the two. He is playing the role of a teenage son who should not coincide with his father, something that has not yet happened with Iván. Usually, in interviews, teenagers have been just as strong as Dani, but much kinder in their ways. A good example is Aitana, who has a reputation for being very direct and yet she has a hard time getting started… until she warms up and shows herself exactly as she is:

Interviewer:"Well, Aitana. Your fame precedes you. It seems clear that you are going to tell me that adults do not have the right to speak like teenagers do. What do you think?".

Aitana (14 years old):"Well…" (nervous laughter. His sister Ainhoa intervenes to recommend that he speak as if he were speaking to his father).

Interviewer:"Imagine that I arrive to class, I see you nervous and to calm you down I tell you: 'Hey Aitana, de chill, okay? De chill'. What would you think?"

Aitana:"Wow. I turn around and say: What's wrong with this one? Let him modernize in his age, not in mine" (laughs).

Interviewer:"So you don't think it's okay for me to correct you like that. I would have to tell you something like: 'Miss, sit down and be quiet.'"

Aitana:"So better".

Interviewer:"And don't you think that speaking to yourself in the first way can break down those barriers that separate students from teachers? Can more trust be generated between both of us?"

Aitana:"No".

Interviewer:"Why not?".

Aitana:"Because he is giving them trust as if he were their friend, and the teacher is not a friend, he is a teacher. It is not his place to speak like this."

Interviewer:"Very good. And if, for example, you talk to your aunt (Thaly, 29 years old) in private, to tell her something intimate, and your aunt uses some of your slang words in that conversation, would you allow it?"

Aitana:"My aunt would allow it. She still has a young face."

Interviewer:"And your uncle Borja?" (Borja Núñez,… older).

Aitana:"If I went to Borja…(laughs) too, too."

Interviewer:"So what is the maximum age at which you would allow an adult to speak like you teenagers do?"

Aitana:"Well…"

Interviewer:"Your sister Ainhoa is close to 18. When she is, will she no longer be able to speak like she does now?"

Aitana:"Yeah. I think that up to 20 you can. Around there, approximately."

Interviewer:"Okay. Well, thank you very much for your collaboration."

Aitana:"You are welcome".

As we see, Aitana is blunt with the teacher's example, but leaves the door open to the possibility that, as adults, we can talk to a teenager using their slang. Of course, only if that adult is considered close, close to them. But what does it mean to be close to them? Aitana is not able to clearly define an age range that allows us to know who is close to them and who is no longer close. For his sister, she calculates the limit at around 20 years old, but for his 29-year-old aunt, she continues to allow these licenses naturally. Even with Borja, who is well over thirty, he is able to tolerate her use of him.

To shed some more light on this matter, we decided to interview

Thaly, Borja Núñez's partner and Aitana and Ainhoa's aunt. Could she explain to us why her nieces don't veto her? This is what she told us:

Interviewer:"Well, Thaly. You are, let's say, in the middle of the two generations. You are an aunt and you are already well over twenty, but you are still considered a person similar to today's kids, as your nieces claim. Why do you think this happens?"

Thaly:"It seems very strange to me, because I don't understand even half of the words they say. I mean, everything is because they explain it to me but I alone wouldn't even understand their Slang."

Interviewer:"Even if you don't know her. When you show interest in her slang, do you think they don't care, that they might even find it cool?

Thaly:"I think so, but only if I do it with them. If your parents ask, they don't like that so much, talk to your parents about it."

Interviewer:"Come on, let's see. We have both of them here. Does that answer seem correct to you?"

Aitana and Ainhoa:(Ainhoa speaks for both of us). "Yes, very correct."

Interviewer:"And why are you not ashamed with your aunt but with your parents? What can differentiate one thing from another?"

Aitana and Ainhoa:(Ainhoa continues speaking). "Because she's not a mother yet. "My parents are already my parents, but my aunt is outside of what they are."

Thaly:"Do you understand?" (laughs).

Interviewer: "Yes I think so. This same thing has come up in other interviews. I think it refers to the different role played by uncles and fathers. Finally, are there any words that you know, that they have told you about this last batch? Something new?".

Thaly:"If you wait. The thing about not kissing each other on the mouth yet, what was it like?" (Aitana comes to her aid and confirms that she means being boque).

Interviewer:"Yeah. To be boque is to be still a little green in love, right? Well, so you know that in the social networks chapter we included this term. You can investigate it there (laughs). Hey, thank you very much for your collaboration. A pleasure".

Thaly:"Thanks to you".

As we intended, the conversation with Thaly, in which Ainhoa and Aitana participate, sheds enough light to be able to draw a second conclusion: the veto is not so much a question of age as of the role with which they perceive the adult: if for them it is a authority figure, such as their parents or teachers, Slang is prohibited. If, on the other hand, he is someone who can be severe at times, but has a role more of advising than sanctioning, like the one that empathetic uncles can play, then he is allowed certain licenses.

The Slang exists precisely to begin to define themselves as adults, breaking with those who until now have shown them the way. How can we know who we are if we only do or say what our elders have told us? That their authority figures, parents or teachers, want to penetrate that necessarily sacred space for the purpose it has, represents a violation that they are not willing to tolerate. Therefore, if we are their parents, it is good to know their slang to get to know them better, but it is not good to use it in our relationship with them. Forcing the situation means violating the trust they have in us. We have another role, they demand it from us. And exercising it is the best way to show them that we will always be there.

However, if we are concerned about teenagers in our environment over whom we do not directly act as an authority figure, it is good to know and use their Slang so that, taking advantage of the exceptional trust they give us, we can influence them positively. With our example, with our own experiences, and knowing how to express them, we can help them understand and understand each other. That they tolerate us speaking like this means that they open the doors wide to their world, that they trust and support us, and that they love us very much.

The interview with Ainhoa, a 16-year-old teenager, left open another door to the possibility that, as adults, even being seen as authority figures, we could interact with teenagers using their slang: joking. According to Ainhoa, if the context is clearly light-hearted, an adult can play at being young again, acting like young people today. These were her words:

Interviewer:"Hello, Ainhoa. You have to answer me if you think that adults should not talk like teenagers."
Ainhoa:"And how do we teenagers talk?"
Interviewer:"Well, with new words, your Slang. For example, if Borja were well dressed right now, could I tell him that he looks is

fachero and that his drip is cool?

Ainhoa:"Nooo, not at all."

Interviewer:"And why not?".

Ainhoa:"Because he's not our age. We must have respect for our elders."

Interviewer:"But if an elder wants to talk like that, why don't you respect us and allow us to talk like that?"

Ainhoa:"Because your time has passed. You already had your time and your words. Now it is the turn of another generation."

Interviewer:"And in some context do you think it would be good for us to talk like that?"

Ainhoa:"Jokingly yes, but in a serious conversation the facherito doesn't look good" (laughs).

Interviewer:"Very good. Thank you so much for the interview. With this you have already given us plenty of material."

Ainhoa:"You are welcome".

What Ainhoa tells us is something that I had experienced in class and I was happy to see, after speaking with her, that it was not poorly received by the students. But as a teacher, there are moments depending on the context, in which we clearly have to be authority figures and others in which it is convenient to relax that profile and appear closer, which could condition their response. Could that be happening? To rule it out, the best thing was to talk to a real authority figure: the mother of teenagers.

To capture this point of view, Sonia, the admirable woman with whom I share this adventure of becoming parents, was willing to collaborate with us, and she told us the following:

Interviewer:"Well, Sonia. You are the mother of three children, one of them, a lost teenager and another, with a very fat pre-adolescence as well. What do you think we should do? Should we approach our children by speaking like them or do you consider that this can be a barrier that separates us even a little more from their world?

Sonia:"I don't think it's necessary for us to speak their language to be close. Although it is true that as a joke, when we are joking, it is fun to tease them a little with that Slang. But other than that, I don't think I should talk like them."

Interviewer:"And not speak, but…know their slang? Do you think it can be a useful tool for you as a mother?"

Sonia:"Yes of course. (He laughs when he sees that she relaxed her gesture after confirming that what we have been saying throughout the book coincides with what she thinks.) That is very necessary to be able to know how they express themselves, what they think, what they say… because if not, we would be very lost."

Interviewer:"Very good very good. If you discover a word that may have risky connotations, how would you approach that conversation with your child?"

Sonia:"Well, in mother mode, in serious mode, I would first sit down and talk to him to find out what he said and why. And then, well, we would see if that conversation can be treated with good vibes or not."

Interviewer:"Okay. Thank you very much for your cooperation. It has been a pleasure. I will continue seeing you at home. See you later".

Sonia:(He laughs without saying goodbye).

Sonia seems to confirm Ainhoa's words, so a third conclusion can be drawn from both: adults, even as authority figures, can use adolescent slang as a joke. This statement is more important than its simplicity tells us. On the one hand, it is essential to keep the communication channels open so that our teenage daughter or son can use them when necessary or when we consider that we need to have a serious conversation with them. Maintaining a relaxed relationship, in which the generational war is fought cordially, between imitations and jokes, greatly favors the possibility of having an important, serious or intimate conversation, when circumstances require it. The use of Slang is, in this sense, a good tool, because as Ainhoa and Sonia tell us, it is well received by both parties in a relaxed context.

But, in addition, the embarrassment that adolescents feel when listening to an adult speak their Slang is a very important resource for working with heterogeneous groups of adolescents, such as those that can be found in any classroom. Nowadays, teenagers are very afraid to open up, to express themselves, to be themselves. It is normal, it would have happened to any of us in this era in which the slightest error can be recorded, reproduced and viralized until it leaves a painful mark, difficult to heal. One of the biggest challenges that teachers have in managing groups is to unite them to achieve an environment of trust in which each one can be themselves, without fear of the other, and grow together from their own characteristics. And one of the tools that work best for me to create that climate is to subject myself, myself first, to that ridicule in public, based on bad jokes, personal anecdotes of blunders and, above all, using many of their words in a way exaggerated, as if he were one of them, but making the pantomime evident. Honestly, I don't think they can be asked to expose themselves if the person who should lead that group does so from the comfort of their teacher's desk. A teacher has the ability to relax the environment, avoiding disrespect or loss of authority. He has tools to allow and cut what he considers necessary until weaving that relaxed atmosphere, in which faces begin to be distinguished from the mass. When laughter becomes widespread, when it is observed in the teacher's flesh that failing is part of learning, that making mistakes is the most natural way to understand what is demanded, learning becomes more significant. And the students and the teacher are much happier.

Finally (and fortunately), a fourth conclusion is drawn from Sonia's words, which confirms the purpose of the book: knowing teenage slang is very useful for getting to know teenagers. Understanding his decisions, knowing his tastes, empathizing with his fears, alerting ourselves to possible risks... in short, continuing to share his life despite his adolescence, helping him when he needs it, even if he does not verbalize it, and enjoying it, enjoying it a lot, because in less Whatever we realize, one day he will go to bed as an adolescent and wake up as an adult.

Conclusions from psychology

Being a teenager is not easy, they live halfway between a child and an adult, fear and the need to know, dependency and the search for autonomy... and in the midst of all this confusion, their slang is perhaps the symbol of social identity. most important thing they have as an age group.

At this point, it is clear that talking about the difficulty of communicating with a teenager is not a surprise to anyone present, and although the ultimate goal of this book is not to delve into communication strategies, I wanted to briefly summarize the importance of the knowledge of the Slang that we have exposed to carry it out successfully, just as we work on it in therapy. At the end of the day, what we sow in the five or six years that adolescence lasts will significantly mark the path that communication with our children will have for the rest of our lives.

Don't get me wrong, love, attachment and respect have been worked on since early childhood, but the perception of "you can talk to my father/mother"somethingthat will make them share important things with each other in the years to come.us, is generated in this period, and is determined by how we have handled ourselves in what we could divide into three large blocks of communication (following the criteria of my colleague, the psychologist D. Antonio Ríos):

1.   Affective

Teenagers are the ones who start the conversation to talk to the parent. It usually happens at the most inopportune moment (once again denoting the impulsivity experienced in adolescence), but there is no option to postpone the conversation, it is now or never. And we can't miss it!

This is when the teenager will express his feelings, emotions and concerns. Knowing the lingo during this dialogue is essential. If we interrupt them with questions to clarify what they are telling us, look like we don't understand them, or ask them to speak like an adult, the conversation will have ended at that very moment. We just have to try to relax and listen actively, even if it is difficult for us to understand everything.

2.   Effective

On this occasion, we are the parents who address the children. It happens when we need to convey an important message, and for it to come to fruition with an acceptable success rate, said message must be clear and brief. There is nothing more fruitless than a sermon at these ages (and I would dare say that almost none).

Teenager slang doesn't come into play here at all. The adult should under no circumstances try to use it. It has, therefore, no greater validity than that provided by understanding the "hidden gift" in the return message, which gives usthey will editreluctantly when they do not share our opinion.

3. Superficial

Don't let the name fool us. It is by far the most important form of communication, in terms of quantity and quality, that should exist between parents and adolescents.

Dealing with everyday topics, without apparent depth in the message, such as talking about hobbies, sports, music, fashion, tik-toks... is what will bring peace to our home, transmitting a feeling of relaxed coexistence, well-being, cohesion or at least , the truce between the parties, so fundamental for the family's daily life.

In this case, again, knowing the teenage slang, both the one they use to express themselves and the one that describes the world around them (games, music, social networks), will play an essential role if we want to understand their world and share relaxed moments. Although each party must have its well-defined role and its own way of speaking, living this "interwar period" will make our children understand that we are accessible and that we can maintain a fluid one-on-one relationship with them, giving them value as individuals. autonomous, moving away from the paternalistic conversations of when they were children.

That after adolescence, our sons and daughters continue to consider communication with us as the main tool of information, guidance, criteria and opinion, it will only be possible if during those years, we knew how to plant that seed of fluid, daily and relaxed conversation.

With these conclusions from experts, both for being protagonists of adolescence and for being psychology professionals, we conclude this book. We hope we have shed some light on your role as parents of teenagers. We are convinced that they are doing wonderfully well, although sometimes you feel, we feel, lost or overwhelmed. In those cases, don't be tryhards, trust yourself, you are pro. Act con la calma, take it as de chill and take advantage of the hype, otherwise you will have FOMO for having missed this wonderful stage.

Teens' detectives at your service:

If you have any suggestions, recommendations or want us to investigate and write about a specific topic, contact us through:

Email: teensdetectives@dobletinta.com
Instagram: @teens.detectives
Publisher: www.dobletinta.com

We greatly appreciate it if you help us with a constructive review on Amazon.

GLOSSARY:

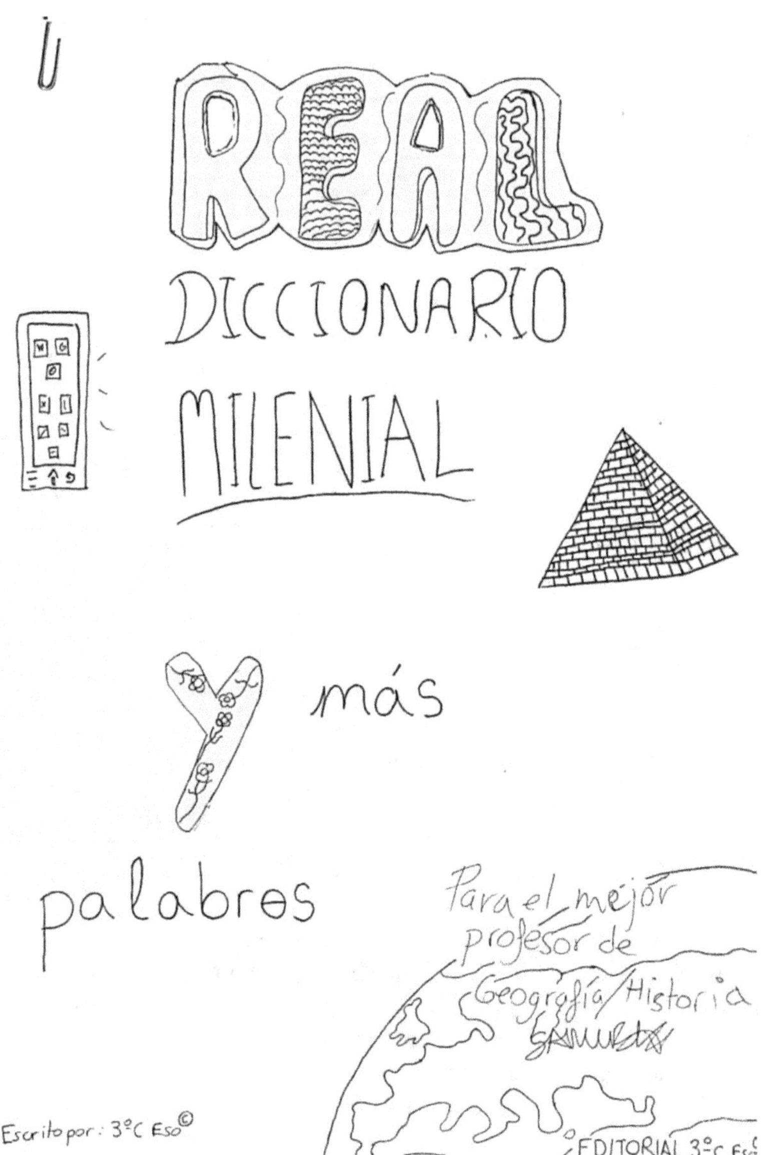

Gift from 3rd ESO students. Class of 2019. It all started with them.

Terms used in adolescent slang.

+1: It is equivalent to "like". That is, it serves to recommend content or recognize your interest.

1-Up: An extra life.

01, 02, 05…: It is the way that young people indicate their year of birth and, therefore, refer to their age. For example, 01 would be 2001.

1174: See you at the party (with wild party connotations).

121: It means chatting privately.

1S1K: Acronym for the English 1 Shot 1 Kill (one shot, one death). Kill an enemy with a single shot.

420: Relating to marijuana and its consumption.

53X or CU46: We meet to have sex

9, CD9, Code 9: The parents are nearby.

99: The parents are far away.

A3: Anytime, anywhere, anywhere.

Adds: Additional monster summoned by one you are fighting.

Aegyo: It is a term used to describe cute and playful attitude or behavior. Some K-Pop idols display "aegyo" in their interactions with fans.

Aesthetic: This term can be translated as visually attractive. It is used to define a type of aesthetic that always seeks to exalt beauty, regardless of the field.

AFAIK (As far as I know): AFAIK; as far as I understand

AFK (Away From Keyboard): It is used to indicate that you will be away from the keyboard or "Not Available", in the middle of a video game or chat conversation.

All in: It refers to betting everything you have on a single bet, usually in the context of gambling.

Ana: Anorexy

ASAP (as soon as possible): Translate "as soon as possible." It can be used in conversations like "I need that information asap."

Bae: An affectionate way to refer to your partner, close friend or someone special in your life. It comes from "before anyone else."

Ban. From English ban (forbid): Blocking access, generally to a service or an online game server. Having a ban or Being banned means having access to a service, server, forum, game, etc. blocked.

Banker: Selection of a bet in which you have a lot of confidence and is combined with another riskier bet to increase the profit.

Bankroll: The amount of money a person has available to bet or play.

Basic: This adjective is used as a kind of insult to refer to something or someone that is boring or not cool.

Beef: Originally, this word was only used in the world of hip hop or trap. Nowadays, its use has extended to everyday speech and refers to the hints that two or more individuals give to each other in a confrontational tone. It can also be used when the fight is physical. Beef originally referred to the rivalry or feud between rappers, often expressed in song lyrics. Now it is used in a broader sense, to refer to any type of discussion or enmity.

Betting the farm: Gambling a large amount of money, similar to gambling one's farm or part of one's estate.

Bias: This term refers to the favorite member of a K-Pop group. Fans often have a "bias" within a group, meaning they have a favorite member.

Binge: Also known as "binge-watch." Habit of binge-watching multiple episodes of a television series online.

Bling-Bling: Refers to expensive, flashy jewelry and accessories, often worn by rappers and Hip-Hop artists.

Blue boogers: Snorting Adderall or Ritalin.

BN: The abbreviation of "Good."

BoA Bind on account: An in-game item linked to your account.

BoE Bind on equip: An in-game item that you cannot trade after you have equipped it.

Bookie: Betting house.

Bots: An AI player controlled by the computer; It is sometimes used as an insult referring to new and unskilled players.

Boomer: Technically, they are those people who were born between 1946 and 1964. However, members of Generation Z use it to refer to those people who do not understand their codes.

Boque: The expression being a "boque" or "un boquerón" is a colloquial expression used by Generation Z, which refers to a person who has never kissed someone. It has a derogatory connotation that describes a person's lack of experience in romantic relationships.

BRB (Be right back): I'll be right back.

Bro. Abbreviation of "brother": It is one of the terms that young people use to refer to their friends or colleagues.

BTW (By the way): By the way.

Buged: Colloquial expression to indicate that a game or a part of it has bugs (errors) that prevent its correct functioning.

Buff / Debuff: A buff adds powers to your character; A debuff removes powers from your character.

Bussing: This other adjective means "very good", "incredible" and is normally used with food, as in the following recipe titled bussing.

Callejero: It is a term used to describe Reggaeton's approach to life on the street, the experiences that occur there and that are reflected in its songs.

Camp: Camping.

Camping: From English, camping (camp). In multiplayer games, it is a tactic that consists of remaining motionless at a strategic point on the map that is difficult to access or has poor visibility, waiting for other players to appear in line of fire to shoot them. It is a very frowned upon strategy and is even penalized on some servers.

Carry: Derived from Carry. When a player "runs" it means that he has enough skill or power to make his team win on his own.

Cash: Available balance in a betting house.

Cast: From English cast (throw). Cast spells.

Caster: From the English caster (caster). Character or player who has the ability to use magic or ranged attack spells.

Cayetano: Term popularized on social networks to refer to what was previously called 'posh', that is, young people from a wealthy social class who like to be dressed in clothes from famous brands and at high prices.

CB / OB CB – Closed Beta, OB – Open Beta: They are both games that you can try before they are released properly.

CD Cooldown: The recharge time after using a special power.

Chalk: Bet with a high probability of being successful.

Chasing: It means continuing to bet or gamble in an attempt to recover what has been lost.

Chetado: Said of a player who is using cheats (tricks) to have an advantage in the game.

Chicken: In shooting games or shooters, a player who dies too many times.

Chill / chill out: This verb means to relax, calm down, rest.

Chinese Farmer: Vulgar way of referring to people who dedicate themselves to playing many hours of online games in exchange for a salary, or other compensation such as room and board, in order to raise characters to a certain level, generally to the maximum level, so that later These are sold to players who do not want to invest the time necessary to level up a character.

CID: Acids and drugs

Comeback: In K-Pop, a "comeback" does not refer to a return in the literal sense, but to the release of new music or a new album by a group or artist. Comebacks are often exciting times for fans.

Counter peeking: From English to peek (take a look) and counter (against). In first-person shooting games, the action of repeatedly peeking out (to seek vision of the rival at a crossfire angle) and returning to cover, taking advantage of this moment to return to shoot.

Cray / cray cray: This shortened version of crazy means something that is out of control or that has gone out of someone's head.

Craft: From English craft (to elaborate). Make objects from existing ones or from basic elements collectible in a game. It is a very common skill in role-playing games.

Cringe: It is an Anglo-Saxon term that has become popular worldwide thanks to the internet and social networks. It is used to describe a reaction of embarrassment or discomfort in a specific situation or behavior. Alludes to moments that are embarrassing or difficult to watch.

Crush: Translated from English, it can mean "to crush", "to fail" or "to crush", but in the language of love it adopts another definition: "platonic love" or "crush". This meaning is the most used in social networks. Therefore, a crush is called a sudden infatuation that is deeply passionate, reveals, excites and excites, regardless of whether it is feasible or not, as if it were a spell.

Dayger: Party during the day

De Chill: The word 'chill' comes from English and translated into Spanish means "cool". It also refers to relaxing or something being "relaxed" or "calm." The term has actually been used for a long time among gamers, to make their teammates understand not to move so fast or to calm down their actions within the game. In addition, "chill" has been part of other popular phrases, such as the famous expression "Netflix and chill", which is used on social networks to indirectly talk about a sexual encounter. Now, apart from all its previous uses, the word "chill" is once again used as a synonym for a joke when users say "it's from chill" or "from chill." In this way they make the other person understand that they should not take what happened personally, because it is just a joke and they should not get angry. It is usually accompanied by the emoji of the little hand with a surfer pose, a hand that has only the thumb and little finger extended.

De locos: Way of indicating that what is being talked about seems fantastic to you, you love it.

Debut: It is the moment when a new group or artist is officially presented in the music industry. It is an important moment in the career of a group and its fans.

Demobow: It is the characteristic rhythm of Reggaeton. It is a repeating drum pattern and is an essential part of reggaeton music.

DIY (do it yourself): Translates "do it yourself." It is seen more on YouTube and Facebook.

DM (direct message): Direct message. It is commonly used on X (Twitter) and other forums.

Dog: Bet on the underdog.

Dope: It is used to describe something that is great, incredible or impressive.

Dospa: Share a joint between two people. Getting involved with two different people in the same night. Go out in pairs of two.

Dupe: From the English dupe (to deceive). Taking advantage of an error or glitch in the game to obtain successive duplicates or clones of an item, to use it indefinitely or to sell it.

DPS: Damage per second: A calculation of how much damage per hit you deal and how fast you can attack.

Drip: This adjective is also used to describe clothing or a sophisticated and modern look. TikTok users upload videos showing their outfits and often use this word in the titles.

Dungeon: A closed area of a game with powerful enemies and great rewards.

Dura/Duro: In Reggaeton, "dura" or "duro" is used to describe someone who is brave, strong or talented. It can refer to a person or a song that is perceived as powerful.

Dutching: Divide an amount of money between several options of the same event to diversify the risk.

El Alucin: El alucin is a term that refers to the altered state of consciousness caused by drugs. However, among young people it is used to describe someone who likes to appear to have a lot and show off more than they really have. It is now beginning to be used in a broader sense, to describe any person who usually tells a notable number of lies.

Epic / Epicity: It comes from epic, that is, great or out of the ordinary, in reference to a game, game, specific action, etc.

Era: This term became popular on TikTok where it is used both humorously and seriously. For example, if you are in that phase of improving as a person, of taking care of yourself, of thinking about yourself, you are in your healing era.

Evens: Bet even or odds 2.00, with which you get double what you bet.

EXP/XP: Experience points: The points you earn for completing tasks to increase your character's level.

Extra: Extra is another adjective that translates to dramatic or likes to attract attention.

F: Expression that has its origin in the game Call of Duty and is used as support or empathy towards someone facing a difficult moment or to express sadness at the difficult moment itself.

Facts: When someone says facts, it means that the information is a fact, a reality and the opposite cannot be denied.

F2F: This is an offer to video chat or meet in person (face to face).

Fachero: Person of good taste, who cares a lot about grooming and dress. It can also refer to an object or situation to indicate that something is attractive or fun.

Fail and Win: Translated it would be "Failure and Success". It is used to express emotion or mockery at the failure of another.

Fan: This term is widely used to describe someone who is a passionate fan of a popular artist, group, or television series.

Fan Service: It refers to the gestures or actions that artists perform to please their fans. This may include close interactions, gifts, greetings, and other loving gestures toward fans.

Fanchant: It is a choreographed chant that fans perform during live performances to show their support for the group or artist. "Fanchants" often include members' names and other specific verse.

Fandom: It is a community of fans who share a common interest in an artist, group or franchise. For example, the "fandom" of a Pop band.

Filch: Similar to camping, being hidden or camouflaged, aiming at your rival from afar to try to kill him.

FYI (For your information): For your information; so you know.

Flamer: Term used to describe the person who is dedicated to insulting and creating controversy with the aim of igniting a conversation. Similar, therefore, to troll.

Flex/Flexin: It is used to describe the display of success, wealth or confidence. "Flexin'" is the act of showing off or showing off.

Street flow: It refers to a style of Reggaeton that focuses on themes related to life on the street, fighting and overcoming obstacles.

Latin Flow: It is used to describe the style and influence of Latin culture on Reggaeton music, characterized by vibrant rhythms and dances.

Flow: It refers to the style and way an artist presents themselves in a song. Each reggaeton player can have their own distinctive "flow."

FOMO: The "Fear Of Missing Out" is the fear of missing out on an exciting or relevant experience. Teens can feel FOMO when they see their friends doing something fun and they aren't there.

For real: With this phrase we ask the other person if they mean what they just said.

Freestyle: It is the action of improvising lyrics or rhymes on the spot, often in an impromptu rap competition.

Fresh: It is used to praise something that is new, modern and elegant. In Hip-Hop, "fresh" is often associated with style and fashion.

Function/Func: Party

G2G (Get to go): I have to go.

Gank: Do ganking.

Ganking: Acronym for Gang Killing.

Gatekeep: In this internet era in which we live, sharing is beautiful and whoever doesn't do it will be said to be doing gatekeep. That is, it refers to those people who do not share information, such as where they bought a t-shirt or where they took that cool photo.

Get rich quick scheme: A plan or idea that promises quick and significant profits.

GG / Goodgames: Congratulations to another player at the end of a game.

Ghosting: The expression "ghosting" someone is used when a relationship with another person, whether romantic or friendship, is suddenly broken. There are different types of ghosting, but, in general, the person who "ghosts" another person decides to stop communicating with them from one day to the next.

Glow up: Referring to a positive transformation from the past to the present. It may be a change in appearance, confidence or personality.

GNOC: It means "get naked in front of the camera."

Go lacasito, go doraemon, go tinkiwinki: basically, he/she is drunk.

GOAT: The acronym stands for "Greatest of All Time," which is used to refer to someone who is the best at what they do, whether in sports, music, or another area.

Green: Term used to refer to dollar bills (in English).

Grind: Spanishization of the English term grinding (to grind, to crush). Killing enemies repeatedly with the sole objective of accumulating some reward, such as experience to level up a character or some equipment or materials.

GYPO: It means "take off your pants."

Hater: Derived from the English to hate (hate) / hater (he who hates). Player who systematically despises, destructively criticizes or defames a game, genre, brand, platform, etc.

High roller / Whale: A person who bets large amounts of money.

High: Indicates being drugged or under the influence of a substance.

Hit: It is used to describe a song or movie that becomes very popular and successful.

Homie: It is an informal term used to refer to a close friend or colleague. It is very common in Hip-Hop slang.

HTH (Hope that helps): It is used when you share useful information with another person and say "I hope it helps you."

Hype: Get overly excited about something. It is also used to describe something or someone that is in fashion, although it is expected to be temporary.

IDK (I don't know): It is used to express ignorance about something.

ILY and ILU (I Love You) and (I Love U): It is short for writing "I love you."

IMO (In my opinion): In my opinion.

Influencer: It is a person who has a large presence on social networks and who can influence the opinions and choices of other teenagers. This applies to Pop music figures and other content creators.

IRL (In real life): With this acronym it is expressed that what is being told is not an invention.

It's giving: This expression is used to describe that something or someone gives you good vibes. It is usually used to praise or highlight something.

Jackpot: The largest possible prize in a game of chance.

Jai: Get high.

JK (Just kidding): It refers to the fact that what was just said is "just a joke."

K or KK (Okay): Okay; OK

Kappa: Emoticon or meme used at the end of a sentence to indicate that it is ironic or sarcastic, commonly used on the streaming platform Twitch.

KDR/KR Kill-to-death ratio/kill ratio: is the number of enemies you killed compared to the number of deaths you had.

Kilometer: In Argentina, synonymous with interrupting, spoiling, bothering, etc. in a game.

KPC: Keep parents off guard.

Lache: Synonym of "cringe", that is, embarrassment of others. Although it can also be translated as disgust or even laziness, depending on the context.

Lag: A network or processing delay that slows down the response time of your game.

Laged: Equivalent to "having lag", that is, having such a great delay in communication with the server and/or the rest of the players in a game that it becomes very difficult or directly impossible to play an online video game correctly.

Legit: Something legit means that something is very good. It is short for legitimate, which means authentic or real.

Light Sticks: are light-up devices that fans bring to K-Pop concerts. Each group usually has their own official "light stick" with a specific design that fans wave during live performances.

Lick: From English lamer (in computer slang, an ignorant person). Performing actions typical of a lick, that is, behaving stupidly, cheating or annoying others, and ultimately in a state of ignorance about the correct way to play.

Lightstick: They are light-up devices that fans bring to K-Pop concerts. Each group usually has their own official "light stick" with a specific design that fans wave during live performances.

Lit: It is the abbreviation of "literally" or "literally", used to highlight the literal meaning of what is said or to make the interlocutor see that you agree with what is said. It can also be an expression used to express that something has a value. very positive for the speaker, that is, as a synonym for "great" or "excellent."

Literary: From English lit (illuminated). Used mainly in shooting games, a teammate is called "liteado" to finish off an enemy who has been injured after a confrontation.

LMIRL: Let's meet in real life

LMK (Let me know): Let me know.

LOL: Acronym for League of Legends, a MOBA-type online real-time strategy video game developed by Riot Games in 2009.

LOLZ Similar to LOL: It is used to express laughter out loud, to point out that something is very funny.

LYKYK (if you know, you know): You know what I mean.

Lyrical Genius: It refers to a rapper or artist with an exceptional talent for creating intelligent and creative lyrics.

MDLR (or mdlr): It is the abbreviation of Mec de la rue, a French term whose translation would be "street boy." It has been made popular among young people, in part, by singer Morad, a 23-year-old artist born in Spain and of Moroccan descent who describes himself on his Instagram account as "MDLR Ni madero ni chivato." In his songs, he talks about what life is like in a working-class neighborhood, loyalty between friends or the difficulties of getting ahead. This term is used among young people to refer to boys from working-class families who have been on the streets since they were very young, looking for a life for themselves and their family. Sometimes it is used in a derogatory way, to criticize an aesthetic considered 'cani', characterized by usually dressing in tracksuits or sports clothing and non-sports accessories, such as chains, rings or bracelets. Other times, MDLR is used as a way to express the fight against any type of social discrimination.

Maknae: The "maknae" is the youngest member of a group. This term is used to identify the youngest member and is often shown affection and protection by the other members.

Manco: Extremely bad player, due to inexperience or lack of playing ability.

Mía: Bulimia

Mic Drop: It refers to a dramatic gesture in which someone drops a microphone after giving an outstanding performance, often used as a powerful final statement, in which there is no right of reply.

Molly or X: Ecstasy

MOOD: It refers to the mood to do some activity. It is seen in expressions like "I'm not in the mood."

MOS/POS: Mom/dad are watching (looking over their shoulder)

M.P/Magicpoints: allows you to perform magical abilities.

Nap: Maximum confidence bet made public by a professional forecaster.

Netflix and chill: Originally, this referred to watching a movie and spending time together, but now this phrase can also be a proposition to have sex.

Nerf: A game update that limits the power of a powerful weapon or ability.

Noob: From English newbie (newbie). Derogatory way of referring to a rookie, generally for not respecting older players, or for not improving over time.

NPC: NPC stands for Non Playable Character. Although its origin is found in video games, it is commonly used on social networks to talk about people without their own opinions, who do not think for themselves or who behave in a predictable way. It can also be used, although to a lesser extent, to refer to people who are in the background, not very relevant in the life of the person making the mention.

NTR: Acronyms for "don't even scratch yourself". Used to express that there is no need to worry or give too much importance to something in particular.

OMG (Oh my God or oh my gosh): It is used to express amazement.

OP: In "Original Poster" forums (or original author). That is, the one who creates the topic being talked about. In gamer Slang, Overpowered: a weapon or ability that is disproportionately powerful compared to other elements of the game.

On fleek: When something is "on fleek", it means that it is perfect or impeccable. It is often used to describe well-groomed eyebrows or well-applied makeup.

Padrear: Padrear is used when a person says or does something that provokes tremendous admiration at a certain moment among his audience. It can be used in the first person when one wants to show off or act cool. Now, those attitudes are called "parenting."

Panas: Group of friends.

Parlay: Combined bet in which all predictions must be correct to win.

Party favors: It can refer to drugs or substances consumed at parties.

Penny Ante: Betting small amounts of money, often on casual games.

Periodt: It is used to settle a phrase that one believes can hardly be refuted. Its origin comes from the word "period" (period, in Spanish). Some users indicate that, with the 't' added at the end, the aim is to place more emphasis on the pronunciation.

Perreo: It refers to a sensual dance style that is often associated with Reggaeton. The dance involves provocative movements, almost always performed by women, and is very common at parties and video clips of this musical style.

Pharming: The act of going into medicine cabinets to find drugs to get high.

Pick: Forecast.

Picket: If for the Royal Spanish Academy, a picket is a wound made with a sharp instrument or a group of people trying to impose or maintain a strike slogan, for young people this word is also synonymous with 'flow', that is, style. innate. You can say, for example, "The clothes are bought, but the picket is not."

Ping: The measurement of time in milliseconds between the player's console/computer and the host server.

Playing the odds: Betting based on the odds of winning.

Playlist: It is a list of selected songs that are created for a specific occasion, to share with friends or simply for personal enjoyment.

Plug: It is used to talk about someone who can get drugs or illegal substances.

POV: It is the English acronym for point of view. It comes from cinema and is commonly used on social networks. It is used to show the way we react that we have or would have when something happens to us, telling it, therefore, from a personal point of view.

Prendio: In the context of Reggaeton, "prendio" or "prendida" refers to being excited or enthusiastic. It can be used to describe a lively party or an excited person.

PvE Player vs.Environment: When you fight a non-player enemy.

PvP Player vs Player: When you fight another player's character.

Rager: Big party.

RAID: Team quest, usually in a single dungeon, including important boss encounters.

Random: This word can be translated from English as "random" and used to refer to something coincidental, that has not been planned. It can also be used when something is strange, which generates strangeness.

Rat Boy: Young person, generally pre-adolescent, who tries to appear rude, despite his or her young age, through shouting, insults and generally hostile behavior, which is usually extremely noisy, exaggerated and tiring.

Ratio: It is used to express disagreement with a comment made on networks, usually on X (Twitter). Many users respond directly to a publication by putting a "ratio" to express that they do not like anything and disagree or suggest others "ratio" certain messages.

Red Flag: A "red flag" is a warning or alarm regarding a type of attitude or behavior that is not appropriate for a person, such as jokes that border on disrespect or attitudes that are not appropriate to the context.

Rent-free: With this adverb we indicate that something has become an obsession, that we can't stop thinking about it.

Rekt: From the English rekt, vulgarism of wrecked (crushed, destroyed). Rekt or Get Rekt is a vulgar expression, common among young people and adolescents, to provoke the player or the opposing team, as a synonym for "We are going to crush/destroy you."

Relax: small party

Rent: That it rents you, means that the result compensates you.

Rizz: This term is often used as a shortened version of the word charisma. When someone has rizz, it means that someone is seductive, has self-confidence, has something that makes them attractive.

Risky business: It can refer to dangerous or risky activities.

Roast: Informal English expression that means "to make fun of." Making a roast on YouTube consists of making a video reviewing some of the insulting comments that your haters make to you.

Robo-tripping: Consume cough syrup to get high.

ROFL (rolling on the floor): Hilarious.

ROI (Return on investment): It is the indicator that measures the success of a tipster.

Roleplay: Role (role, function). Play according to the rules and characteristics of a role-playing game or simply play a role-playing game.

RT (Retweet): Forward a message on X (Twitter).

Salseo: Any controversy or controversy carried out on social networks that users like to comment on.

Selfie: It's a word that has become ubiquitous in teen culture thanks to the practice of taking photos of oneself.

Set: Synonym of camping, or camping, also with negative connotations.

Shippear (Ship): It refers to the action of supporting or desiring a romantic relationship between two fictional characters or two celebrities, often from Pop music. It comes from the term "relationship" in English.

Si soy: It is an expression used to indicate that one feels identified with a publication or a situation. Thus, simply, it is the response given after the situation raised by the interlocutor.

Skin: A cosmetic change to your character's appearance.

Sksksk: This expression is an onomatopoeia used to represent laughter, often in situations that are funny or adorable. It is sometimes combined with "and I oop", which comes from a viral video where someone interrupts themselves while speaking.

Slay: Used to praise someone who has done something exceptionally well or who looks incredibly good. It can refer to the way someone dresses or how they perform a task.

Slaying: When someone is "slaying," they are dominating or having great success at something, whether it be their appearance, attitude, or achievements.

Sliving: This term devised by Paris Hilton means living your best life. It is the combination of two words: slay (which would be translated as "hit it" or "make it great") and living.

Sloshed: To be drunk.

Smash: Have casual sex.

Speed, crank, uppers, Crystal, or Tina: Methamphetamine.

Squad: It refers to a close group of friends or colleagues. It is commonly used to describe your social group.

Stacks: It can refer to piles of money or chips in a gambling game.

Stalking: It comes from the English word stalk and means gossiping about the profiles of other users on social networks, whether famous people or anonymous people who have piqued your interest.

Stan: The term "stan" is derived from the Eminem song "Stan" and has become a word used to describe passionate and dedicated fans of a group or artist. To "fan" someone means to be a loyal fan.

Stomp: From the English to stomp (to stomp very hard). Win an online game decisively.

Stream: It refers to the action of playing music or online content, which is common among teenagers to listen to their favorite songs.

Sugarpic: is the request for a suggestive photo.

Swag: It refers to someone's personal style, confidence and attitude. In Hip-Hop culture, having "swag" is a desired quality.

Taunt: From English to taunt (to mock). Make mocking movements to provoke the opponent and try to get him to make an attack movement. Very common in fighting games.

TBH (To be honest): Sincerely; in fact.

TBT (throwback Thursday): "Memory of the past". It is used to remember an old publication or photo.

TDTM: Talk dirty to Me.

Thank you, next: This colloquial term was popularized by the singer Ariana Grande and her song titled in the same way. It means "thank you, next" and means that something or someone was useful, but no longer.

Thank you, next: This colloquial term was popularized by the singer Ariana Grande and her song titled in the same way. It means "thank you, next" and means that something or someone was useful, but no longer.

Their: An abbreviation of "suspicious" or "suspicious." Teenagers use it to describe something that seems strange, questionable, or worthy of suspicion.

The 'jennys': Way of referring to girls who, like the MDLR, like to dress in tracksuits and other sports clothing, accompanied by non-sporty accessories such as large hoop earrings, rings, etc. Before, the term 'choni' was used more, but as has happened with 'posh', it has been replaced among the new generations by 'jennys'.

Throw Down: To have a party.

Throwback (TBT): It is a term used to refer to something from the past, such as a retro song or fashion. Teens often post photos and memories as part of "Throwback Thursday" (TBT) on social media.

THX (Thanks): "Thank you". A quick thank you.

Tipster: Sports predictor that recommends bets to other users.

TL;DR (too long; didn't read): Too long, I haven't read it.

Torch: In the context of teen slang, "tea" refers to gossip or interesting, current information about people's lives. If someone says "spill the tea," it means they want you to tell them the gossip.

Trap: It is a subgenre of reggaeton that often features darker and more thematic lyrics that they call "street" lyrics. It combines elements of Reggaeton with Hip-Hop influences.

Trend: It is the way of expressing that something is trending. Tik Tok virals are also called that.

Troll: Person who posts messages that are generally provocative or offensive in chats, forums, social networks, etc. with the sole purpose of generating controversy or annoying the rest of the participants in the community.

Tryhard: Perfectionist player who invests a large amount of effort and concentration in carrying out a strategy in the game to win it or to achieve an objective that in many cases did not require that amount of effort, and who suffers if everything does not go as desired.

Turnt: It is a term used to describe someone who is excited and ready to have fun at a party or event. It can mean "to be high."

Tusa: It is a word that means sadness or disappointment in Reggaeton slang. The song "Tusa" by Karol G and Nicki Minaj popularized this term.

Twinning: It comes from the English term "twin", which means "twin" and in social networks it is understood as dressing the same as another person. Until now, that had negative connotations, as it was an embarrassing situation. However, it is something that is now celebrated and even provoked by being fashionable.

Vape/ Vaping: Referring to the use of electronic devices to consume substances, often nicotine or THC.

Vibes: The word "vibes" refers to the sensations that a situation, a context, a place or a person gives off in the subject. It can be with positive or negative connotations, talking about good vibes or bad vibes.

Viral: It is used to describe something that spreads quickly online, such as a song, video, or trend.

Visual: It is the member who is considered the most attractive or aesthetically pleasing in a group. This term is often used to describe the member who is seen as the most handsome or beautiful.

Wasted: It refers to being very drunk or high.

White lady: Cocaine, heroin.

WTTP: Do you want to exchange photos?

X2: It is used to express that you agree with a comment said previously. If someone else has already used it, you can say "X3", "X4", etc.

YAAASSSSSS: It does not have a defined number of A or S and is another way of saying "yes", but with a lot of enthusiasm.

YOLO (you only live once): You only live once.

ABOUT THE AUTHORS

N. De la Puerta (Madrid, 1981) has a degree in Geography and History. He has worked as a secondary school teacher since 2004 and currently participates in various educational projects that seek to promote healthy coexistence at school.

Borja Núñez (Madrid, 1988) has a degree in Psychology. He has worked in the training and psychological support of young people who are preparing to be sports professionals. He is currently part of a Family Guidance Center where he helps families with problems derived from adolescence.

Together, they form a professional team that, from their respective fields, from their extensive experience and from the proximity of working daily with adolescents, is capable of taking a critical and accurate look at the risks, fears and problems that concern the fascinating stage. of adolescence.

Together they form, therefore, Teens' detectives, a discreet and in-depth investigation at the service of mothers and fathers of teenagers.